Rescripting Family Experiences

Experiences

The Therapeutic Influence of
John Byng-Hall

Dedication

This book is dedicated to and forged from the very deepest and truest love for Joel, Kirsten and Lauren and the invisible web of my family – but paramountly to Kate, the very first among equals, my existential soulmate. All have schooled me in family life, helped to make secure the base, and been able to say together 'oui' to the joy of life.

Rescripting Family Experiences

The Therapeutic Influence of John Byng-Hall

Edited by

JOHN HILLS

Family therapist, Canterbury

W

WHURR PUBLISHERS

LONDON AND PHILADELPHIA

© 2002 Whurr Publishers
First published 2002 by
Whurr Publishers Ltd
19b Compton Terrace, London N1 2UN, England and
325 Chestnut Street, Philadelphia PA, 19106, USA

British Library Cataloguing in Publication Data
A catalogue record for this book is available from the
British Library.

ISBN 1 86156 263 2

Contents

Foreword

It is a gift to have a serious and deeply insightful book that refracts a life as a good prism does a complex light source. The colours making it up are fanned out and displayed and we are treated to reds blending into oranges and on and on. When they recombine we know the light differently.

John Byng-Hall is a friend and colleague. I have known him, without exception, as a man of sweet candour, unflinching in telling the truth as he sees it, with a deep sense of the tragic complexity of life that has led me to always feel safe in his hands. While I have known the stories about his life that appear in this book, after reading it I realized I had not really known them at all. As I turned each page the dramatic tension came close to being unbearable: it seemed I was reading with a hand at my throat.

Biographers tell us about the life and work from the outside in; autobiography comes at it the other way, from within outward. In family therapy these holographic projections meet at the family script – as they do, we learn in this volume, in the best of theatre. And, in the best of therapy.

The autobiographical account of John's boyhood years in Kenya, his crippling illness with polio, the brutalities and nobilities of his medical education, is fascinating, harrowing, and finally illuminates not only his life, but our lives and our work. It is in the end a redemptive account, redemptive, as he tells us, in that the telling allowed him finally to bring into the same story, the image of his athletic self next to the disabled self.

Coherence and wholeness are as close to expressing the goals we seek and it was in search of these that John began the autobiographical writing that became the kernel of this volume.

We have also much about psychological theory and the practice of psychotherapy, with particular emphasis on the areas of John's special interests; attachment theory and family scripts. These sections have been written by colleagues and students out of their interest in him and his work.

He emphasizes the elements in his own story that provided the fertile ground in which his interests flourished. Thus, the book in its construction, by including this history and theory of the family therapy field as well as the account of John's life, becomes an isomorph for the stance it takes about family scripts. Here is the work; here is the life. The same paradigms rule: we co-create what we observe, the stories about their families we propose to tell to our patients and the multiple nuances with which these conversations are constructed is who they, and we, are.

A brief concluding lament: family therapy (or systems practice) of this quality, the interest in theory, the spaciousness of viewpoint, has these days become more and more of a rarity in the US, where I live and practice. I was fortunate to be among the first wave of American family therapists washed up on the UK beaches in the early 1970s, to work with John and Rosemary Whiffen and a dozen other wonderful colleagues who became friends and now repay the favour by being our teachers. This volume could not be produced in my country these days. I note with gratitude that it has been created elsewhere.

Donald A. Bloch, MD
February, 2002

Preface

JOHN HILLS

> Suffering must needs be borne twice; once in the body and once in the soul.
> (Sophocles, *Oedipus the King*)

Psychotherapy is a formalized enabling dialogue between at least two people centring on the exploration of meaning and better living within the personal experience of at least one of the participants and for which the relationship between them may form part of the basis of the conversation. 'Therapeutic conversations are organised by the desire to relieve mental pain and suffering and to produce healing' in the view of Canadian family therapist, Karl Tomm (1988).

Family therapy, as a therapeutic method, was started tentatively and experimentally by John Bowlby in London in the immediate aftermath of the Second World War. He invited whole families into a therapeutic conversation and began to harness the multiplicity of relationships and different members' perspectives in the exploration and healing (Bowlby, 1949). In doing so, the method broke absolutely with Freud's central psychoanalytic stricture that the therapeutic conversation was solely between patient and therapist (Freud, 1917). Since then, the family therapy movement has adopted this ethos of experimentation and extending boundaries to produce a whole harvest of fresh ideas, methods and techniques in antithesis to traditional psychotherapy approaches.

Such approaches usually assert a single road to change which can only be achieved through strict adherence to their particular method. Family therapy, however, in its respect for and celebration of diversity, has always pursued a pragmatic restlessness, synthesis and eclecticism in its active quest for therapeutic change. Corey and Bitter (1996) provide one of the most succinct accounts of this developmental history and the many different strands and boisterous voices. Not only is this in part a reflection of the outlook of one of its early thinkers, the polymath Gregory Bateson, but also of the rapid adoption of systemic thinking, a process analysis that explores the connections between difference, and in doing so creates a new synthesis. Family therapy has a remarkable ability to draw on current ideas in the sciences, social sciences and humanities: thus social constructionist, deconstructionist, feminist and postmodern currents of thought are all present in the field, in the service of examining the intersubjectivity of human relationships in a way unrivalled in psychotherapy. Sometimes this has also meant that the emotional depth of therapeutic work, the strength of many traditional approaches, has been sacrificed for brevity and innovation.

These many modifications of approach to family therapy over the last 55 years have made for a rich mix. Sometimes, however, they may have left some of its practitioners and trainees with a certain breathless bewilderment at its inclusivity. Although the defining principle of family therapy has been the active inclusion of significant family members, with true commitment to the process of circularity there has now developed a growing corpus of work with individuals (Asen and Jenkins, 1992; Boscolo and Bertrando, 1996). Family therapists in the UK now prefer to be known as 'family systemic therapists' or, simply, 'systemic psychotherapists' to indicate the emphasis of systemic ideas over those of family in their approach. Many who do not wish to be identified specifically with psychotherapy, but who prize the use of systemic ideas in their work in the human service professions of social work, nursing, medicine, clinical and educational psychology and counselling, etc., prefer the designation 'systemic practitioners'. The UK professional association for family therapists is now known as the Association for Family Therapy and Systemic Practice. So what is the nature of this systemic understanding?

Systemic thinking is generically understood as a way of examining the structure and pattern of organization (from the ancient Greek *systema*, from *syn* — 'together' and *histanai* — 'to set'; thus 'to set together'). The Greeks used this concept in their political thinking to mean 'organized whole'. Whatever is, has pattern, process, structure, organization and interconnection. This may be inorganic such as climate, the geology of our planet, indeed, the cosmos itself; or organic, e.g. the botanic and zoologic; or the human structures of our physiological, sociological, psychological, ethnologically constituted worlds. Our whole universe is composed of multiple organized patterns of intricate interconnecting systems with complex cybernetic (from the ancient Greek *cybernetes*, the steersman) mechanisms for self-sustainment. This is the totality of our ecologically situated being and of our systemic existential nature. We are also self-aware, experiential beings, governing and governed by the impingement of different systems of which the intimacy of personal, family, friendship and work-based relationships are the most immediate and substantial. It is for our experiential self and these systemic relationships — the subjective and intersubjective realities — that psychotherapeutic help is often sought.

As different systemic schools have developed, what has been considered as forming the organizing pattern and the *domain of experience* has changed. There are more frequent crossovers with traditional psychotherapies than are sometimes acknowledged. Early in the history of family therapy, emphasis was placed on the emotional life of the family, incorporating psychodynamic understanding of the interplay of conscious and unconscious conflicts. Later a cybernetic perspective was used to explore problems and symptoms, as an enantriodromic tension between the opposites of change and stability which trapped the family in restrictive, repetitive, feedback loops.

A consensus has always been maintained on the importance of the family lifecycle in activating change. There followed, in no particular historical order, focus on the experiential domains of: family structural boundaries, hierarchies and the distribution of power — the politics of the family; the cognitive life of the family, its different beliefs, assumptions and perceptions of one another; solutions, problems and life strategies; the communication between family members — language, gesture and the interpretation of different levels of meaning; the behavioural, action-reaction feedback pattern; narrative, the family's selective capacity to promote and demote accounts about itself and its resourcefulness. More recently, in the confusingly named 'second order cybernetics', feminism and postmodernism there has been a return to an examination of the subjectivity of the therapist's own beliefs and a questioning of the assumption of an observable objective reality. The therapist's perception, cultural beliefs, gender assumptions and ideas about difference which might act as a source of therapeutic distortion, dominance and experiential dissonance were all subjects for exploration.

These are the component elements of the process analysis of systemic therapy, and how the family embodies and is configured in these domains of experience is the total process which may be called the family script. However analysed or synthesized, it is the template for helping to understanding how a personal and intersubjective experience is organized as well as how the therapist is located in relation to the process.

Systemic psychotherapy may be seen then as 'conceptual Esperanto' — though hopefully with a wider usage! — that seeks for a universal 'language' to give meaning and coherence to diversity in relationships and experience. Its relationship to psychotherapy could be compared with that of Hinduism to religion: a highly flexible, inclusive framework of diverse forms with a huge pantheon of 'deities' and beliefs (some very localized, others universal) which is able to incorporate into itself ideas from other religions. In comparison, traditional psychotherapies seem exclusive and monotheistic, dedicated to fixed beliefs. Just as Hinduism is deeply rooted in the cultural experience of India, so systemic work is rooted in the cultural experience of family relationships. Each shows a remarkable capacity for tolerance, adaptation, assimilation and colour.

Rescripting family experiences

This book, *Rescripting Family Experiences: The Therapeutic Influence of John Byng-Hall*, like all offspring, has developed a life of its own quite different from my earliest expectations — and is all the better for it. Originally I had intended to draw on a number of contributors from very different fields in the social sciences and psychotherapy, who, familiar with John's work, would examine the idea of the family script from their particular perspectives. This would have been true to the spirit of John's work as an integrator. He has always valued the metaphor of the bridge and much of his work is just that — a bridge between family therapy, psychoanalysis, attachment theory, ethology, drawing, painting, child and adolescent mental health. This would, however, have tipped the balance towards an academic discourse and away from an experiential and practical workbook for family therapists at all levels of training. Other psychotherapists, interested in John's work or curious about what is going on over their family garden fences, might also be engaged. This book was never intended as solely a valediction to John. I wanted to include work in progress by family systemic psychotherapists influenced by him, who may have taken his ideas in other directions and so would help the book to do what John does best — stimulate new connections and renewed awareness.

As the book developed, John offered a much more detailed and reflective autobiographical account of his life. This gave the book a very different turn and sharper experiential edge. It is then, in a phrase beloved of soccer commentators, an event of 'two halves'. The first part belongs to John and to Rosemary Whiffen, co-leader of the first family therapy training course in the UK at the Tavistock Clinic, London.

The first chapter is his own narrative. John wrote recently (Byng-Hall, 1997) that 'narrative' to 'therapy' is as redundant an expression as speaking of a 'tooth dentist'. It is the more surprising then that family systemic therapy has yet to produce an autobiographical equivalent of, for example, Jung's *Memories, Dreams and Reflections*. John's personal narrative goes far deeper into this unwritten territory than any systemic psychotherapist I have read to date. The story engages the reader fully and reveals the congruence between John's ideas and their basis in experience. It is difficult not to read it without feeling both moved and inspired by his personal struggle, and his reflections on the act of narrating. Here is the genesis of the elements that make the striving for integration and acceptance in the face of adversity, disappointment and personal distress. To make available to others what has been garnered and understood on that journey is to transform the base metal of personal suffering into the elemental gold of healing. This is the psychotherapist's art; this is the journey Sophocles intended his audience should understand from the Oedipus scripts (Sophocles, 429–420BC), rather than the narrower meaning psychoanalysis has disseminated.

John Byng-Hall has wished to preserve the privacy of his own family of creation and, while highly significant in his own development and having their own perspectives, these do not form the core of his very personal account. Perhaps this is the basis for another book!

Though personal therapy has never been a formal requirement for the training of systemic psychotherapists, extensive self-reflexivity and live supervision are. (This may explain the absence of autobiographical accounts.) John's account of his family of origin, his childhood, young adulthood and early career development may challenge the wisdom of this and certainly will stimulate greater self-exploration.

What follows is a conversation between John and his colleague, Rosemary Whiffen (Chapter 2). The story of the formation of their landmark course within the fiercely psychoanalytical culture of the Tavistock Clinic, the largest National Health Service psychotherapy training centre in the UK, is important to the recorded history of family systemic therapy. Their gender and professional equality as course leaders — one a psychiatrist, one a social worker — was an important affirmation of the importance of joining difference and helped to create a context in which the early course tutors — Caroline Lindsey, David Campbell, Ros Draper and Gill Gorrell Barnes — could develop.

The second half of the book consists of five very different accounts of work in progress from psychotherapists with whom John has been closely associated either as colleague, trainee or supervisee. David Campbell traces his own emerging professional identity and its subsequent diverging pathway within the Tavistock family systems training (Chapter 3); Jeanne Magagna, on her journey of integration between Kleinian-based child psychotherapy and family systemic psychotherapy, helped by John (Chapter 4); Sara Barratt examines the context of working in GP practice and the unique continuity such a setting provides for understanding family relationships and the impact of family scripts(Chapter 5); Kate

Rescripting Family Experiences

Daniels explores the interface between script in the theatre and in family relationships, two professional worlds in which she is familiar and between which she comfortably moves (Chapter 6). Finally, the editor takes a philosophical tack by exploring the existential context and importance of the human family and its defence against death (Chapter 7).

In each chapter, the experience of family-life-script and relationships, real or fictional (family members in the former are given fictionalized names to safeguard confidentiality) is described and explored. Family systemic therapists do not create scripts in their work; their work is more analogous to script editors, drama coaches, directors, interpreters and critics. They are also simultaneously audience and observers, as in the ancient Greek chorus. Their own scripts are both enabling and disabling; the expertise comes from knowing the difference.

John Byng-Hall's contribution to the development of family therapy has been substantial and significant. He taught me a great deal of what I know; and to know where to look if I do not. Though he has retired from the Tavistock Clinic he has not retired from practice. It is to him, the past work he has encouraged and inspired and the work as yet uncreated, which will bear his influence, that this book is both tribute and appreciation.

Acknowledgements

I have appreciated a great deal of help in the preparation of this book from many sources: my thanks to John Byng-Hall and the contributors for their patience in the redrafting process; to East Kent Community Health Care Trust for allowing some flexibility in my working time to complete it; to Robin Royston, consultant psychotherapist and clinical lead, a highly supportive colleague; and to my other colleagues at the Adult Psychotherapy Department at Cossington Road, Canterbury for their humour, support and encouragement. To Julie and Jean for helping with the typing. To Mary Godden, wise counsellor, for our wide and varied conversations. The children, families and colleagues at Heath Farm Family Services, Charing Heath, Kent and ISP, Sittingbourne Kent for all their input to my learning and understanding over ten years. My gratitude is undying in all sorts of ways to Kate Hills whose incredible stamina, editing and production skills make *Context* magazine such a vital part of the UK family systemic practice community and who really pulled out all the stops (and put in some to improve the text!) in gathering this book together.

I would like to acknowledge and express appreciation to the estate of Louis Macneice and to Faber and Faber for permission to use 'The Truisms' from 'The Collected Poems of Louis Macneice'.

This book was written before the events of 11 September 2001 and their aftermath. These are the accelerated moments in history when the sense of what it means to be a family is particularly heightened and challenged, across all cultures; when the effect of loss and dislocation has to be rescripted into many family experiences.

This has truly been a labour of love by everyone involved, and like all love it has had its moments of doubt, but this has never succumbed to the burden of the labour.

Introduction
Telling one's own story: from farmer to family therapist

John Byng-Hall

Prologue

I am writing this for myself. Why? I began to review my life after retiring from the Tavistock Clinic in the autumn of 1997 and what strikes me when looking back on my life is that there was a complete disjunction between my childhood in Kenya, which was largely outdoor, active and farming, and my adult life in England, characterized by disability, cities, medicine and psychotherapy. The contrast is intellectually understandable in view of my having polio at the age of 18, which forced a dramatic change in what I could do as I entered adulthood, but to me it remains something of a puzzle as to how I became a very different person. I cannot put the image of myself as a child or adolescent and myself as an adult comfortably within the same frame. I do not have a coherent story that allows me to see how I made such a transformation.

Semi-retirement seems to me to be a good time to reminisce or, perhaps I should say, it is difficult not to reminisce. I now have a four-day weekend and have time to contemplate my past. I am also becoming more disabled by what is called post-polio syndrome, in which there is further loss of muscle 30–40 years after the initial paralysis and overstrained joints give way. Not surprisingly my reminiscing turned to the first illness when I was 18 and what that meant for me.

Many years ago I gave myself a rule that if I proposed general theories about people then they must have some relevance to myself and therefore I should purposefully explore the issue within my own experience. I have always followed this rule by looking at how various ideas that I had written about have been played out in my own life. But I haven't yet applied this rule to helping families to tell a more coherent story about themselves, and their past. Mary Main's attachment research showed that the capacity to tell coherent narratives about past attachments is associated with greater security in current attachments, and with a reduced likelihood of developing problems (Main et al., 1985). One of the questions asked in their interviews was how do you see the past influencing how you are now?

I need to explore how my past led to my present. I have set myself some rules before writing:

1. I will write a story that makes the journey from childhood to adulthood.
2. This will be done in one steady stream without making edits during the process.
3. I will write it as if I am telling the story to an interested stranger who does not know the story already and would not pass it on to anyone else. This is to ensure that I will not leave out any major part, however personal. The aim is to write a story to myself, while recognizing that a story's power comes from sharing something with someone else, in this case with my inner confidante who can also tell it back to me in written form after the telling.
4. I will keep a diary about how I experienced the writing.

Later

I have now read my story. I personally found the whole process powerful and very fruitful and I can now see how my past led to my present. So I decided to share my experience with other family therapists in case it might be useful. For this purpose I have chosen to select only those aspects of the story that throw light on what it was in my past that led to me becoming a family therapist. As a trainer I had explored this issue with students using a family tree. They have often told me that that exercise had been fruitful. Using a similar way of telling oneself one's own story might hopefully provide one way that family therapists can do this for themselves.

I have omitted any details of my current family as sharing details about them is inappropriate.

Chapter 1
My story: why I became a family therapist

JOHN BYNG-HALL

Part I: Kenya

Childhood: danger and beauty side by side

My first memory was of a snake slithering along my pram towards me, then veering away and sliding up and over the side. Was it a memory or the product of my imagination or many images woven into one memory? Who knows? It is real enough in my mind, but it is hard to accept that it all goes back to my infancy in the pram. However, we did live in Kenya where snakes abound. The pram was often left under the eves of the thatched roof of the garage – a common place to find snakes. At one time a family of fat overblown puff adders took up residence there. Cobras, black mambas, green mambas and many other poisonous snakes lived around the house. But the image I have is of a slim brown striped snake; it was probably a harmless grass snake. I was always frightened of snakes nevertheless. When I went to the lavatory, which was twenty yards from the house in a small round thatched hut, I would first look down the pit to see if there was a snake curled up on a wooden ledge a couple of feet below the seat. I would then gaze up at the roof until I left. I never told my parents, or my sister who was 18 months older, about my fear. Nor can I remember any of them telling me about their fear. That was my family.

Most of my later memories of snakes were of seeing them in the grass. A particularly vivid image was of cantering on my horse and becoming aware that a black mamba, head held high above the tall grass, was weaving its way at incredible speed – as only a mamba can – alongside the horse. Luckily it veered away – perhaps this contributed a strand to my 'early memory'. Quite frequently we would hear the Africans shouting '*Nyoka! Nyoka!*' (snake) and gathering together armed with sticks to beat the snake to death. The main story my parents told me about snakes was of

1

being woken up by the African cook who told them that there was a curious noise coming from the wireless. A spitting cobra was found curled around the valves, a nice warm place for a snake. Woken up, it proceeded to spit its venom into the eye of the cook: a very painful process and dangerous for sight unless dealt with quickly. My parents poured some milk in his eyes. After about three days his eyes were better and he could see again. This story was used as instructions for what to do if it happened to someone we were with. If no milk was available then water would do. But if caught out on the plains without water it was better to use urine than wait until reaching water supplies.

Above the lurking dangers of the bush the world was strikingly beautiful, even to the eyes of a child. We lived, isolated, on the floor of the Great Rift Valley in all its spectacular splendour as it cut a vast furrow through the Highlands of Kenya. Here it was 40 miles across, with lakes and volcanoes along its floor at 6,000 feet, with sides soaring up to 10,000 feet in places. As a child I can remember many times sitting down on a boulder in the middle of the plain and gazing at the sides of the valley in a daydream in which I felt merged with the immensity of its space. In the rainy season I became fascinated by the huge cumulous storm clouds towering to well over 30,000 feet, their white fluffy tops appearing in the distance over the edge of the valley. The clouds slowly revealed their full immensity as they came over the side of the valley; their heavy black bellies darkening the forests beneath, only broken by brilliant flashes of forked lightning and almost continuous rumbles of thunder. I watched as the cloud's shapes slowly changed, hinting at mighty spirits, thousands of feet high, lurking in their folds. As the storm approached the trees became people, dancing as they twisted and turned in the gusting wind. Eventually the glorious rain hid everything in sheets of life-giving water. I was peopling the valley with my fantasies of both dreadful angry power and gifts of deluging proportions. Trees often evolved into dancing 'people' in my drawings. It is interesting that in Africa spirits are often seen as entering trees, although I did not know this as a child.

My sister Caroline and I were brought up in Flamingo House, so called because it lay halfway between lakes Nakuru and Elmenteita in which, we were told, up to half the world's population of flamingo congregated at times. At six o'clock in the evening many thousands of flamingo would fly between the two lakes in V-formations, their long necks outstretched and wings flashing deep scarlet underneath, their characteristic gabbling noise rising to a crescendo as they passed overhead. For me as a child this is just what happened at 6.00 p.m. I nevertheless remember watching them with awe. Was this a young child's sense of beauty stirring, or had I picked up how my parents never ceased to marvel at such a sight?

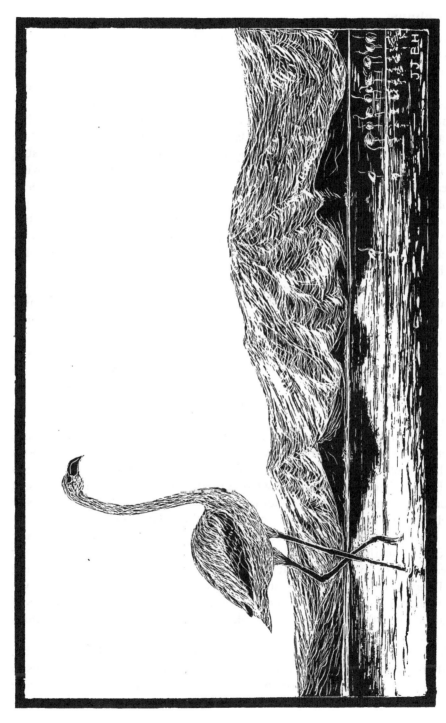

Figure 1.1 Flamingos on Lake Elmenteita with Mt. Eburu beyond: scraperboard drawing by John Byng-Hall aged 16.

My mother

My mother was a water colourist. She would never have seen herself as an artist but she was. She also embroidered some wonderful designs for cushion covers based on the animals, birds and flowers on the farm. She helped my sister and me to draw and paint. Caroline developed a very lifelike way of drawing animals with sweeping bold lines that captured their movements perfectly. When she was 16 Caroline managed to sell a set of scraperboard Christmas cards of African wild animals. For a while they were the most popular cards for sale in East Africa. In my usual competitive way I also sold a selection of scraperboard cards the following year. They were not nearly so good and were drawn with very thin lines so that they could not be reproduced. They never did appear in the shops. We learned to use watercolours, and when I was about 11 my mother taught me to paint in oils. She also taught me to knit and embroider. This was a very rich form of early learning, free of the male stereotype, for which I am very grateful.

Although my mother was talented in many forms of artistic endeavour she had many other roles. She had been a VAD nurse (voluntary) as a young woman and she carried out this role on the farm. Every morning there was a long queue of people waiting for her ministrations. I learned that Africans were incredibly brave. I can remember seeing a man standing waiting patiently with a huge gash that half-severed his foot. He made no attempt to jump the queue. This level of bravery and patience was obviously expected by everyone, otherwise he would have been ushered to the front.

My mother talked to us a lot about people. She was really a city person, interested in social interaction, so she would always be puzzling about why people behaved as they did. After we had visitors she would discuss why they had done and said what they did. We were also recipients of some running comments about our own behaviour, or heard stories she told about us to others. I was learning 'mother's knee' psychology.

My mother described me as being a kind little boy and liked to tell the story about the bald visitor who stayed with us when I was about four years old. My mother had cut my hair just before he came. She was sitting talking to the man who was sitting on the sofa. She suddenly noticed two little hands appear from behind the sofa and solemnly place little pieces of hair all over the man's bald pate. She did not recount what his response had been.

One of my mother's favourite stories about me was about leopards. When I was about five and my sister seven, a leopard killed some calves in a thicket a little way from the house. The next day the family was driving near this thicket when my parents spotted an unusual bird and both got out with binoculars to watch it and disappeared into the thicket. (Their hobby was bird-watching.) My mother told the story: 'After we had been gone a while John got out of the car, found a stick and a stone and came looking for us to rescue us from the leopard. Caroline in the meantime sensibly wound up the windows, curled up on the back seat and read a book.' This story was told to celebrate my bravery. Later when I explored the nature of this legend, I was able to see that it could be interpreted in exactly the opposite way. I was probably frightened and went in search of my parents to protect me. The sticks and stones were to protect myself rather than them. It did perhaps show that there were expectations that I would become a masculine protector. Caroline understandably felt very insulted by this story.

The farm

We lived on a 50,000-acre farm called Soysambu which spanned half the valley floor and one slope. It encompassed Lake Elmenteita, which was 10 miles long and 3 miles wide. The terrain was very varied. On the valley floor savannah plains were separated by ridges covered by thick shrub and cactus-like euphorbia trees. Forest covered the sides of the valley, while there were volcanoes like Mt. Eburu and lava flows to the south. Hundreds of species of birds were to be seen, many colourful and exotic. It was equally rich in animal life: leopard, antelope of many species, aardvark, hyena, monkeys and baboons, and many others. There were 4,000 dairy cows and some 20,000 sheep as well. My father, who was employed as the farm manager, was out most of every day. Milking never stopped and needed overseeing. As we grew older he would take us with him in his car as he did the round of the farm. This was when we saw most of him. He was very kind and rather silent, but we would hear him talking Swahili to the farm workers. As we began to understand more he discussed farming issues with us. This was fascinating.

My sister and I explored the farm on horseback. We would get up at 6.00 a.m. to ride during the coolest part of the day returning at about 9.30 a.m. to a huge breakfast, which was the main meal of the day. By the time I was ten I was exploring the farm on foot with a .22 rifle, keeping the family in meat. At night I would inspect the bedroom for snakes and other ominous creatures and then pull the blankets up over my head, afraid of animals coming through the window. I would lie listening to the many night noises.

Our family was very isolated. As children we were not allowed to play with black children and the nearest white child lived 15 miles away, an hour's drive. My sister and I learned to entertain ourselves, establishing a complex world of our own, inhabited by 'plumsey' men. As these games were elaborated we started to half-believe that they were real little people who lived under and around particular boulders. We built roads linking each boulder. When we had a visitor we would look for a trail of dust appearing in the distance inching its way closer and closer until we could see the tiny speck of the car in front of the cloud of dust. The excitement would became almost unbearable even though we knew it would take at least another half hour before the hubbub of the arrival, with greetings and hugs and suitcases to be marvelled at.

We were only once separated from our parents. When I was about three and my sister Caroline about four and a half years old they left us for a weekend at a children's home where there were many children, a sort of weekend crèche. I can remember my sister and I standing in our cots crying for our mother. Nobody came. When our parents eventually came to collect us I remember sitting looking at a log on the ground and trying to ignore them.

Schooling

My first school was four hours' drive away. My mother had taught my sister and me through a correspondence course during the war but when I was seven and my sister nine, my parents finally decided that we should go to school. My mother started a propaganda campaign to convince us, and probably herself as well, that it was a wonderful idea. I remember becoming quite excited by the prospect. Then at the last moment I was ill and had to go to the doctor. He said that I should go a week later, and clearly expected me to be delighted, rather than disappointed. When the time came it was a terrifying and terrible experience. We had no experience of being with other children and found ourselves being caught up in hordes of milling children, all of whom, by then, knew where to go and what to do. To us it was like being caught in a huge wave, tumbled upside down and round about, to surface we knew not where. No sooner were we beginning to find our bearings when the next wave came crashing down. I had never been separated from my sister before. She went to a girl's dormitory and I to a boy's. I can remember seeing her at the other side of the school hall in floods of tears and feeling very upset for her and not being allowed to go to her. What strikes me now is that I cannot remember expressing my feelings about the terrible betrayal, or crying for my mother. I am sure I must have done so. But perhaps this was when I started to cut off my feelings to protect myself. Perhaps this explains why I can remember seeing my sister's distress better than my own experience.

I may also have become more of an observer of life, less of a participant. I know that my mother became worried that I was too good, to the extent that she went to see the headmaster about it. He knew exactly what to do. He put me in the bed next door to the archbishop's son, who was the naughtiest boy in the school. This worked beyond my mother's wildest dreams: we used to go for 'midnight walks' (probably about 9.00 p.m.) to explore the country around the school in the moonlight. Our favourite excursion took us along the railway line to a place where it became a viaduct. We would then lie down underneath the viaduct and watch the trains passing overhead. It was fantastic. The steam engines were fuelled by wood, so we could see the flames pouring out and sparks flying in every direction framed by clouds of steam. The noise was totally engulfing. The thunderous rhythmical 'chuff chuff' of the steam engine came first, followed by the roar of hundreds of wheels passing along the line, each making a noise like a gun as it passed over the gaps in the rail. The sense of power was overwhelming: the earth shook as the train strained to climb the steep gradient towards Equator station at 9,000 feet before it rolled down towards Lake Victoria. No modern day nine-year-old's viewing of television could possibly compete with the reality of this thousand-ton fire-breathing monster passing a few feet above us, in deliciously forbidden time and place. The danger was real too, the sparks regularly caused fires. But why was I not frightened? Perhaps animals were scary, machines not. Or my friend was fearless. My mother told me later that she knew the ruse had worked when my slippers were found a mile down the railway line. I wonder if she knew how dangerous it had been. Moonlight adventures came to an abrupt end.

The war

I was two when the war started and eight when it finished. The six o'clock news would be heralded by the portentous sound of Beethoven's Fifth Symphony. Adult heads would be shaken as ominous news was announced. It escaped my child's mind that the events were happening many thousands of miles away. To make the war seem very close we were witnesses to almost continuous mock battles. The farm we were on was used as a major training ground for the army and the air force. During the day the 25-pound guns roared away as small puffs of dust, several miles away, showed how close to the chosen target the shells were exploding. Brenn gun carriers raced past, while platoons of men swarmed like ants across the plain below the house. One day they mowed down a pedigree bull that wandered across their line of fire creating an irresistible target. Abject apologies did not allay my father's fury.

During the night a dazzling display of firepower would light up the night sky. An island in the middle of Lake Elementeita was the favourite target. Brilliantly coloured flares would be fired high into the air to hang on their parachutes as they lit up the lake. As they slowly drifted down on to the lake surface the tracer bullets would make a series of red arcs across

the surface of the lake towards the island. The next day we might walk on
the lakeshore and see the debris of the bombardment. On one occasion a
childhood friend came with us and discovered an unexploded mortar
bomb. He turned it over with his toe. I shall never forget the roar my father
let out when he saw this. Later we watched from a distance while it was
exploded. The danger was real.

Suddenly the war was too close to home. My uncle was killed on D-Day.
My mother went into a withdrawn state. She retreated from us to cry and
my father took us to one side and explained that she was very upset and
why. We never took part in the grieving. We never knew him although he
had visited us briefly just prior to the war. He was my mother's much loved
younger brother, who had been a professional soldier since his training at
Sandhurst. He was a 30-year-old major when he died on the beaches of
Normandy. He was much admired by my mother who saw him as the
epitome of dignified bravery. He was a wonderful shot who had won the
first prize at Bisley. I explored the manner and place of his death many
years later on Arromanches beach. It seemed likely that he had been first
out of the beach craft rather than following the usual rules about officers
going last and using the ratings as early cannon fodder. His closest friend
was wounded at the same moment (which was, of course, one way of
staying alive). This friend was honoured by being asked to lead the parade
of 7,000 veterans along the Normandy beaches on the 50th year anniversary 'for being first out on the beach'. It was inconceivable that my uncle
should not have done the same. On visiting his regimental museum I
asked the curator what had happened. He said he was not allowed to
discuss the details, 'But I can say that he knew no fear.' I had something
difficult to live up to.

My parents' stories of the past

My father left school when he was 15. He was a scholar at King William
School on the Isle of Man and already had a scholarship to Oxford. He was
bored having to wait until he could go there. His father was an
Administrator in northern Nigeria and only communicated through
telegrams. He sent one to my father's aunt who was looking after him in
England: 'Have been shot in arm with poisoned arrow. Stop. Will die. Stop.
Send John [my father] to Theo [their brother] in New Zealand. Stop.' It
was not until he was on board ship that my father found out that my
grandfather had recovered. He was delighted about the change of direction in his life, but the school was furious.

When my father arrived in New Zealand he found that his uncle had
bought a small island just offshore that he hoped to sell off as plots of land
to disgruntled army officers who did not want to live in England after the

First World War. He and my father went to live on this island with some cows, chickens and horses. He was able to ride one of the mares – the others were wild and he reported some awkward moments with the stallion. After a while his uncle returned to the mainland and my father was on his own. Being ingenious he built a crystal set with a 30-foot tall aerial which when directed at America was able to tune into a California radio station. This kept him in touch with the world.

He could also ride across to the mainland once a month on the neap tides. One month the weather was so bad that he could not get across, a very serious situation as he soon ran out of food. Luckily he could signal to the couple who were living on the adjacent island who had a boat. They were also in some trouble but they were able to pick him up and they sailed to the mainland. My father had lived his 16th year on this island, most of it on his own. He vowed he would never live on an island again. He went to Australia where he had some cousins who had a sheep ranch. The only story he had about this was that he arrived by train at a small station in the bush to find a large Rolls Royce plus chauffeur waiting. Circumstances had changed. He worked on the farm for a while and learned to shear sheep. When he was 18 he sailed back to England arriving at Southampton in pouring rain and a dock strike. His father, who was on leave, met him and said, 'Well, my boy. What do you want to do?'

'Get out of England!'

'Where do you want to go?'

My father thought for a moment and said, 'I want to go to Kenya.' He had a friend who was just about to go there. My father did not recount any discussion about whether or not he should take up his place at Oxford.

With this friend he bought a farm in the Kitale district of Kenya. He told a number of stories about this time in his life. On arrival he had to build a house. He found an attractive spot in a clearing in the forest, and the Africans built him a small round hut of wood with a thatched roof, in their own style. He woke in the middle of the first night to hear a rustling noise. Looking out he could see that a large herd of elephant was passing either side of the hut and brushing against it. He went back to bed and pulled his blankets over his head. The next day the Africans were not at all perturbed, saying, 'But you wanted your house on the elephant trail.' At another time he and his partner were setting traps for lions who were feeding themselves on their home-grown beef. When out and about he suddenly heard a loud bang and found his leg caught in a lion trap set by his friend. Luckily this powerful spring trap, which closed like a huge set of teeth, had pinned the back of his calf rather than smashing his shin. There followed hours of standing in pain before his friend found him. Another lion story: he was leaving a party late at night following a car on his motor bike when the car slowed apparently to let him go by. As he accelerated past he was confronted by a pride of lions walking across the road. All he could do was to wend his way through the pride; he did not recount whether the lions were equally surprised. Leopards this time: he was woken in the middle of the night and saw a leopard silhouetted against the night sky perched on the windowsill. The next moment it had jumped down and scooped up the dog from under his bed with its huge paw. In a flash it was out of the window with the howling dog in its jaw. Luckily leopards preferred dog meat to human meat. Perhaps this story contributed to the way in which I used to imagine animals coming in through the window at night.

My father got blackwater fever and nearly died. He was told to watch his fingernails and if they went black he would die. Hardly comforting. His father came from Nigeria to be with him.

Things did not go well on the farm. It seemed that the two young men had chosen a place that could not sustain European-style farming. They had to sell up and my father went to work near Nakuru, in the bottom of the Rift Valley eventually working for Lord Delamere at Soysambu. Early on his arrival at Soysambu he was called to go to a place where some cheetah had killed some sheep. As he arrived a cheetah broke cover and ran. My father jumped out and, feeling he had to do something, aimed the rifle in the general direction of the speeding animal and fired. The cheetah rolled over and over, dead. His reputation for shooting spread like wildfire. Very sensibly he did not do any shooting after that, thus keeping his reputation intact.

Home leave

Most British people in Kenya would go on what was called 'home leave' to Britain for several months every four to six years. This was an indication that they identified themselves as British rather than Kenyan. We were no exception. We went twice, in 1947 when I was nine and again in 1951. It was a startling experience for us. The sun was still out at ten o'clock at night. That is all wrong: the sun goes to bed at six o'clock. There are huge buildings. The tallest buildings in Kenya were three stories and there was only one of those in Nairobi. The vast majority were one story high. But in England there were buildings that sailed up into the sky. Churches. What is more when you get inside the ceilings rise to wondrous heights. I became obsessed with churches and cathedrals, and collected many books about them. When I was nine I designed a cathedral. On and off I thought about being an architect, that is until I heard that you had to do a lot of maths.

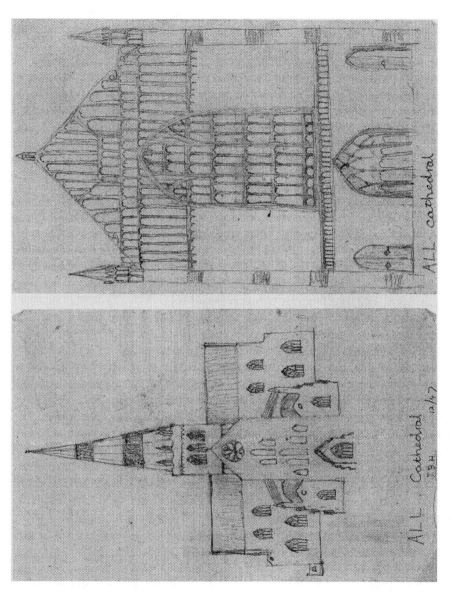

Figure 1.2 Design for ALL Cathedral: drawing by John Byng-Hall, aged 9.

I discovered that I was still anxious about outside threats. In England it was men who might do me harm, and I remember looking out over Tunbridge Wells from a window in my grandmother's house wondering about the people who lived there. Perhaps all children feel anxious and the anxiety will be focused somewhere, depending on their surroundings or their imaginations. As it was my sister and I were mugged (not called that then) by some boys in our street. That never happened to me in Kenya. My mother said that she had been terrified as a child by the idea of a man coming down the corridor with a wooden leg, going clonk, clonk, clonk as he got closer. In the 1947 holiday there was a major polio epidemic raging and we were not allowed to go to the swimming pools. Another thing to worry about.

Adolescence

My family moved to their own farm just as I became adolescent. It was perched high on the edge of the valley. The view was spectacular, looking down into the second largest volcano in the world, Mt Menengai, and up to the other side of the valley 40 miles away. The farm was at 8,000 feet and consisted of a series of steps, the level sections consisting of plains, and some marshes, while the steep rises were covered in thick forest with magnificent 120 foot trees. It was very beautiful.

My mother designed the house and my father built it with stone and wood from the farm. It was on the edge of the forest with a lawn that sloped down to give the house a wonderful view of the valley. Originally the house had been used by the farm's managers, but when we moved in more rooms were needed to accommodate our family. A separate building was constructed some 15 yards from the first. The lavatory, as in Flamingo House, was some way away, requiring a 20 yard walk into the forest. The building that Caroline and I occupied consisted of two rooms, each with its own veranda but not interconnected. In other words, each of us lived in a separate dwelling and had to go outside for everything at any time of the day or night. I found this frightening. It was made worse by the night noises. Small animals called tree hyraxes made a very loud and terrifying noise, like stuck pigs, although we got used to them in time. But there were many other night noises because the forest was full of birds and animals and the crickets were in full cry all night long. We soon got to know the various sounds.

After a year or so I started to hear changes in the forest night sounds – sounds that showed that the animals and birds were being disturbed. At the same time there was an increasing number of reports about social unrest, particularly among the Kikuku people who resented the presence of the colonial power. I became more frightened, and started to spend much of my time watching the open window. There was no way of shutting it properly. I insisted on keeping my loaded shotgun under my bed. My parents appeared to be unconcerned; I felt that I needed to be a sentinel, keeping guard for my unsuspecting family. My parents must have started to worry as well though because they put some iron bars at the windows. However, I cannot remember any discussion about whether or not we were anxious or whether it was wise to be living in this isolated place. Looking back I think my parents, especially my mother, must have worried a great deal but had the notion that if they showed any signs of it we would become anxious. Of course, what happened was that the less anxiety they showed the more I felt I needed to be watchful. Far from protecting us from worry they heightened my anxiety. I worried about my parents' safety while I was at school. I listened anxiously to the radio every evening desperately afraid that it would be announced that my parents had been killed – I was not at home to keep watch and be ready with my gun.

It is hard to remember the exact sequence of events. The news got worse and eventually a state of emergency was declared to counteract the Mau Mau rebellion of the Kikuyu. The armed freedom fight had started in East Africa. As this saga was unfolding my parents made a series of changes in an attempt to make Caroline and me safer. They built a passageway between the two dwellings and put in an indoor lavatory, eventually moving us into the main house to sleep in the dining room. By that stage I had taught myself to keep awake all night to watch the bedroom window, finally allowing myself to drop off to sleep at dawn. Bars do not stop bullets, or spears.

I had become a friend of a Kikuku boy called Cheggi. He looked after our horses, but we also went hunting together in the forest. One day he behaved differently and led the way to a clearing in the forest in which a dog was hanging from a tree. This was a sign of the Mau Mau. I am not sure that I read Cheggi's signal to me that we were in danger; it may have been before it became well known what a hanging dog meant. Cheggi and I, as 14-year-olds, not surprisingly shared some heroes. The son of our white, next-door neighbour was 25 and had just moved to his own farm. He was our hero and we used to discuss him on our hunting trips. One day came the news that he had been murdered. In the stables next morning our eyes met over the back of a horse. It was the most poignant moment of my life. In those few seconds we recognized that we were on opposite sides. We never spoke again. I heard later that he had joined the Mau Mau. It was several years before I could salute him in my mind's eye as having made the appropriate move.

In the early phase of the Mau Mau rebellion isolated farmsteads were attacked by gangs of up to 500 Mau Mau who would advance on the house, shouting and blowing whistles. They would then set fire to the house. One night we heard the noise of a large number of people shouting and whistling, coming closer to our house. We barricaded ourselves in one of the rooms with our guns pointed at the door. This was the most frightening moment of my life. When they came within a few feet of the house, they stopped and fell silent. One man called out. My father immediately recognized the voice of one of the Kipsiggis, a tribe who were opposed to the Mau Mau. He explained in Swahili that the Mau Mau had stolen their sheep and cattle, and that they had come to get help from us. The shouting and whistling had been to keep up their own spirits. The relief was tremendous. We immediately went out and started to search the forest for the Mau Mau. Caroline and I joined in. We might well have been in some real danger at that point, but we found nothing and returned home in the small hours. The next day my mother went tracking in the forest with Caroline and me. We were in hot pursuit when the neighbouring white farmer, whose son had been murdered, caught up with us. He was also on the trail (and unwittingly ours as well). He was absolutely furious with my mother for taking us into the forest. He had been about to open fire on us; he could hear people but could not see properly. Having firearms on your side can be life-threatening.

One day we heard that a couple we knew well who lived quite close had been attacked. The husband died immediately; the wife had terrible mutilations. She was a doctor who was well-known for helping her black patients. At this time it was common for the Kikuku employees to be forced at gunpoint to provide access for the Mau Mau to their white employer's homes. The more trusting the relationships within a household the more likely they were to be targeted. We prided ourselves as having particularly good relationships with the workers on the farm. One day all the Kikuku employees came to the house and waited in a queue. Each came in to give in their notice for assorted reasons, such as a grandparent being ill and needing to be looked after. We took it that they were avoiding a similar position by leaving, and we felt grateful.

All four of us had been armed for some time. It now became necessary to be able to use our firearms within a fraction of a second if someone burst into the room. We practised with unloaded guns: we would take it in turns to go outside and then rush in unannounced giving those in the room practice at shooting at intruders. On one occasion I was the last to burst in and, as the practice was ending, I went to sit in an empty chair. A revolver lay on the arm. I idly picked it up and took aim at my father's back, and then put it down again. Only then did I notice that the revolver was loaded. My father had reloaded it as the practice ended. I came out in a cold sweat when I realised that I could so easily have practised pulling the trigger as well. I still have that feeling of cold dread in the pit of my stomach when I remember this. Up to that time we had had an absolute rule that never, in any circumstances, would any of us point a gun at anyone. The 'practice' broke this rule with near fatal results. I never told any of my family about this. I should have done so because we needed a warning to agree a clear signal to announce the moment of reloading – or to abandon the practice.

The rebellion affected my school life as well. The boarding school that I went to was in the forest, north-west of Nairobi. As the situation became more dangerous we senior boys had to mount an armed guard all night, in three-hour watches, observing each side of the building with our loaded .303 rifles from behind sandbags at each doorway. This was like an extension of my night time sentinel role at home, except that it was official and I was not alone. We were all trained in either the army, or naval or air force cadet corps. I was in the army.

It became increasingly clear to me that we were as likely to be killed by our own guns as to be protected by them. When I was about ten years' old, I had had an earlier intimation of this when I had been unloading a rifle on returning home from a hunt. The bolt slipped and it fired. I had been following the rule of pointing the rifle at the ground, but the bullet hit a stone and ricocheted up past my sister who was coming to meet me – another dreaded memory. The father of the boy in the next bed in the dormitory at my secondary school was killed when his revolver accidentally dropped to the pavement. I heard his son cry himself to sleep over many months.

Am I brave or am I a coward?

Bravery was an issue for me well before the Mau Mau rebellion. I was an anxious boy. My mother once said to me that courage was being able to act despite anxiety – those who know no fear were not truly brave when doing dangerous things. Although this definition helped me feel less ashamed about being anxious, it nevertheless heightened my anxiety about whether I would act in a courageous way when faced with real danger. There were two main scenario in which I imagined being tested. The first was in facing a charging lion, elephant or another dangerous animal. Would I remain sufficiently calm and clear-headed to hit the target, or would I panic or even flee? The other scenario was in war. Would I attack the enemy in dangerous situations or run away? I saw others as being brave, not myself. I would envisage these scenarios many times in my imagination, either in day-dreams or when identifying with someone in the many books I read about hunting or war.

A powerful family legend was told me as a boy. It went something like this. Your great great, etc., uncle Admiral Byng was sent to fight the French fleet off Minorca. When he got there he did not get close enough to the

French fleet to do battle, stayed out of range, and sailed away. He was found guilty of cowardice and shot on his own quarterdeck. Here was a terrifying scenario about the fate of those who run away. There was also no escape from the story, as it was a relatively well-known piece of British history. If my parents had not told me then others would. My parents distanced themselves from this cowardly behaviour by pointing out that the disgraced uncle was the son of a famous and courageous Admiral Byng who had been Admiral of the Fleet. We were directly descended from him and not from the disgraced Admiral. Here was the unanswered question; would I be like one Admiral Byng winning battles or would I run away like the other? The fact that these events took place two centuries earlier was as irrelevant as the fact that the Second World War was being fought thousands of miles away. To me I was there inside the imagery – here and now. Adults tend to forget that a child disappears into a story.

It was not until many years later that I researched the reality of that naval battle. I went to the British Museum to read some of the original documents and found that almost all the legend was untrue. Byng did get close enough to get into range; a battle did take place; ships were dismasted. He was not found guilty of cowardice but only of negligence of duty. I read contemporary accounts of his courageous behaviour in the face of battle. It was possible that he was shot as a scapegoat for the politicians who had acted too slowly to stop Minorca from being taken by the French. I came to the conclusion (1982) that this legend was a cautionary tale about how one should not run away from danger, and that we had been told the story in this form when danger was present. My parents may have used it as a way of bolstering our stance of not leaving the farm, a highly dangerous place. Churchill used the 'shot for cowardice' version of the Byng legend. He had had to persuade the British not to run away when dangerously isolated in the war.

At the age of about nine I decided that I wanted to go into the navy. As we lived 300 miles away from the sea and had no experience of ships, I guess that this might have been as a result of identification with the brave Admiral Byng. About two years later, the HMS *Birmingham*, a Royal Navy cruiser, captained by a family friend, came to Mombasa. I was invited to spend time aboard to see if I liked the navy. One night was enough. I woke early to hear the officers abusing the ratings on deck. It left a nasty taste in my mouth; I had never heard grown-ups treat each other in such unpleasant ways.

Hunting

The gun can be a symbol of manhood. Aged about nine I was given an airgun that fired single lead pellets under high air pressure. It could kill small birds and rats. I was fascinated by the hunt. When ten I was given a

.22 rifle, capable of killing small antelope, rabbits, bigger birds and human beings. Now I could go out in the morning and come home by lunchtime with a dead antelope. Thompson's gazelle made very good eating. I became a good shot and at one time held the school record for a score on the target range. My kudos went up. Within a year or two I was using my father's 12-bore shot gun to shoot partridge and guinea fowl and quail. This was even more fun. Running after a flock of guinea fowl was exciting because they ran fast and every now and then one would drop out of the race and try to hide in a bush, only to fly off when I came close. Halting and shooting as quickly as possible required real expertise.

My mother supported my shooting but my father seemed strangely disinterested. The only time I can remember him shooting, I was amazed that he failed to kill any guinea fowl even though they were sitting in a tree. Many years later I discovered that he had used blanks as he did not like to kill. He gave me permission to shoot because he knew it was important for my self-image. After he had killed the cheetah many years before, he very rarely shot any animals and then only when he had to. For instance, he shot a leopard which had been taking sheep and a rhino that had been caught in a wire trap. The result was that he maintained the reputation of being a very good shot despite not hunting. A very cunning strategy – or perhaps it reflected his aversion to killing – or perhaps it served both functions. The other time that my father was highly successful was on the night that he proposed to my mother. They had been in a boat together on Lake Naivasha and he had been shooting duck in an inspired way. No blanks this time. He must have known that prowess with a gun was greatly valued by my mother because her brother had been such a good shot. It seemed that shooting was a clear symbol of male potency. She knew that in Kenya her son would have to shoot to become a man.

I can remember loving the Geener shot gun, which became mine. It was beautifully made with delicate scroll-work on the stock and part of the barrel. It also shone a dark blue colour. I lovingly cleaned it until it shone brightly when looking down each barrel. It was undoubtedly a phallic symbol during my adolescence. However, I started to become averse to killing antelope when I wounded one, smashing its leg with a bullet, and followed it for miles before being able to kill it. Just before it died a large tear fell from its eye. I can visualize it now and it still upsets me. Birds, unfortunately for them, do not have faces that convey suffering, so my focus shifted to them. I was taught how to hunt properly by one of my father's young managers, Sam. I also had a school friend, Mark, who shot animals more frequently. I returned to shooting animals when in the company of these two people. I can remember, however, being much more excited when shooting birds.

When Mark and I were 18 he arranged for us to go shooting lion. I remember being anxious about this although Mark seemed unconcerned. He had been asked to do this by the farmer who used to shoot a lot of lion but was too busy to pursue a pride of lion that had killed a flock of sheep on the top of a hill. We did not have any heavy rifles but took lightweight rifles more suited to large antelope or zebra. We were not too worried about it as we felt sure we could borrow his rifles. We drove all night because the farm was a long way away, arriving early in the morning. Somewhat to our consternation we found that he had only a rifle of the same calibre as our own. He was such a reliable shot that he could guarantee to hit the lion in exactly the right spot to kill it. A more powerful rifle fires a heavier bullet at high velocity, sufficient to stop a charging lion in its tracks wherever it is hit, allowing for a second shot to kill it. My anxiety went down when the farmer said he would come with us. He took us up the steep road to the top of the hill where the sheep had been killed. Half way up he paused and pointed to a rock and said, 'I was walking up here yesterday and came round the bend and there was lion standing just by that rock (about ten feet away). So I shot it.' He continued to walk as if it was just a passing comment of no particular significance. My anxiety took a sharp leap. When we reached the top he showed us where the sheep had been killed and then took us to the edge of the hill and pointed out the valley where he thought the lion might well have gone. He then said, 'Goodbye, best of luck. See you this evening,' and walked off. My anxiety rose and remained high for the rest of the day. We did go to the place that he'd suggested. I seem to remember, however, not being too fussed about avoiding making any noise when approaching the valley. We saw no lion. The anxiety fell away as it got dark and we had to return to supper. I never learned whether I could stand my ground when being charged. I did find, I suppose, that I could keep going towards danger, even if the locals did not blink an eyelid about doing so.

Physical prowess and risk taking: the transition to manhood

Throughout my adolescence I tested my strength against the elements, often in ways that exposed me to danger. Our school was in Karen, named after Karen Blixen, who wrote *Out of Africa*. It was about 12 miles from the Ngong Hills which were on the edge of the Great Rift Valley, some 100 miles south of our farm. The hills consisted of a ridge seven miles long, with about eight peaks along its length, rising to 2,000 feet above Karen. The other side of the hills plunged very steeply 4,000 feet to the bottom of the Rift valley, an astonishing sight. These hills provided no challenge to climb, they required merely stamina; a 36-mile walk and about 6,000 feet change in elevation if the whole ridge and all the peaks were climbed.

They proved irresistible to young boys, however. There were the vistas and the attraction that they were out of bounds and they extended into the Nairobi National Park, which contained large quantities of game; just enough of a risk to be enticing. At 6.00 a.m., eight 14-year-old boys quietly climbed over the school fence, and returned at 6.00 p.m. We saw buffalo from the top of the hill. They were too far away to be a danger although we might have passed quite close on the way down. The most dangerous moment came when there was a loud hissing noise from behind me and there was a puff adder stretched across the path.

A friend of mine called Peter was an expert in thinking up dangerous wheezes. At the age of 16 he and I planned a bicycle ride down to the coast from Nairobi. This consisted of 300 miles of dirt road, much of it through Tsavo National Park, renowned for its rhino and elephant. The park was set along the base of Mount Kilimanjaro, Africa's highest snow-capped peak that reached to just under 20,000 feet. We planned to camp on the way at Tsavo River. This place was made famous by the book, *Man Eaters of Tsavo*, an account of how a man-eating lion had killed many men who were building the railway. This gave it a particular edge, even if man-eating lion are very rare.

Our parents balked at this, and tried to find some excuse to prevent us going. Illness came to the rescue. My father had to have an operation to remove his gall bladder and was destined to be in hospital for six weeks. He asked me to run the farm during this time. That was even more irresistible, as well as compulsory. I had acquired all the skills to supervise most of the farm functions: driving and mending the tractor, fixing the milking machines, dealing with plumbing and carpentry crises, driving the car down to Nakuru to shop every week. What was beyond me was to take charge of a 50-strong labour force. It was in the middle of the Mau Mau troubles. I found it very difficult to exert the necessary authority. My mother no doubt had the actual authority but women were not supposed to do this. In retrospect, I wonder if I was given the exalted role of managing the farm to entice me away from our dangerous venture. I did take the role very seriously, and it lead to some extremely difficult situations in which my authority was challenged, but I prevailed partly because I was continuously armed, either with a revolver or a shotgun.

Later in the year Peter and I thought up another ruse: to climb Kilimanjaro. Peter had climbed it the previous year on an outward-bound trip, so he knew the way. That was all that was needed in our eyes. We recruited two other 16-year-old boys. Somehow this time we succeeded in persuading our parents. We followed the route, more of less, of the outward bound course. This meant, though I did not realize it at the time, a route that, naturally, provided the greatest challenges. The more usual route from the south followed a well worn track. People did not get lost; most climbers used porters who knew the way. They took five days. The northern route was unmarked, through virgin forest full of wild game. The base camp, which went by the wonderful name of Loitokitok, was at 3,000 feet. When we reached the moorland above the forest at about 11,000 feet we had nowhere to sleep. We eventually found a cave to sleep in. The next day we woke to find ourselves shrouded in cloud. We were completely lost. Luckily we had brought a compass and knew that if we went due south we would eventually meet the track that would lead us up to the top hut at 16,000 feet.

It was raining and so the scree was a layer of thick mud. As we climbed higher the rain turned to snow and we worried that the snow cover could cause us to miss the track. We were just able to make it out and were very tired and extremely grateful when we arrived at the top hut. We were dismayed, however, to find that the door had been left open by the last occupants and the floor was covered by a six-inch layer of ice. Worse still they had also broken all the wooden beds and burned them for firewood. Not good climbing manners. I am not sure how we slept, if at all. This was the coldest I have ever been in the whole of my life. We had to start our final climb at 1.00 a.m. in order to reach the summit at dawn. It was pitch black; we had not thought to plan for climbing with a full moon. We discovered later that we had chosen the one time of the year when the mountain was said to be unclimbable because of the bad weather. It was snowing hard, and the scree was soft below the powdery snow, which made climbing at a 45 per cent gradient very difficult indeed. Undeterred we went on upwards.

As dawn broke we found ourselves at the top of a snow valley whose end was blocked by a 30-foot tall wall of ice. In the darkness we had wandered up the wrong track. We were all now feeling very sick with altitude sickness, which was to be expected at just under 20,000 feet. It was an enormous effort even to stand up, let alone climb. It was clear that we would have to go down a thousand feet, cross over a ridge, and then climb up again to reach the summit that was only a few feet above us. For the first time we made a sensible decision. We gave up the attempt to go all the way to the top and enjoyed the view for a time before descending. The cloud had cleared and we could see over a hundred miles. It was breathtaking.

When we got down to the top hut, the usual destination after the climb, we decided to give it a miss – sleeping another night on ice did not appeal. When we could not find the cave on the moorland we continued down through the forest. It was beginning to get dark, and the game was on the move. Luckily we did not see any. We were, of course, once more

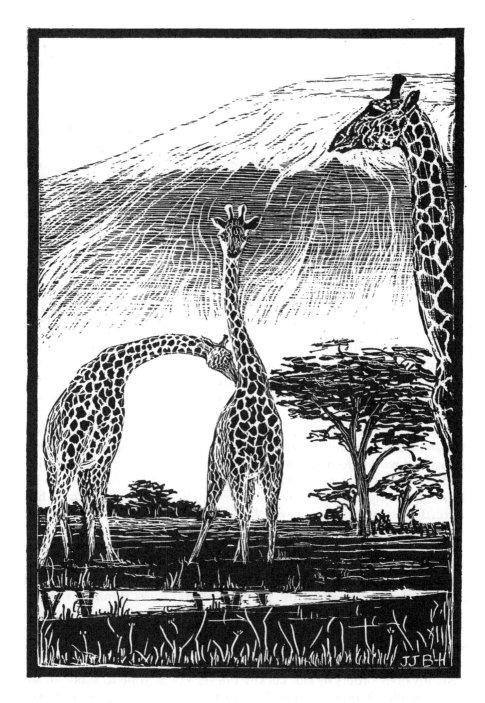

Figure 1.3 Giraffes at the foot of Mount Kilimanjaro: by John Byng-Hall aged 16.

completely lost, but we knew that the road to Loitokitok wound around the base of the mountain and so judged that if we went on downwards we would reach it eventually. We reached the base camp well after dark. When Peter took his boots off he found all his toes were frost-bitten. Luckily he later lost only his toe nails, not his toes.

We had made the climb in three rather than five days. On the last day we had climbed up 4,000 feet and descended 17,000, and were continually on the move for 20 hours, covering some 35 miles. That record, along with its concomitant risks, proved an important test of being a strong fearless male. Accounts of the shear stupidity of the whole venture were blended into the telling of the story, again and again, to give it humour, but more importantly, it provided an aura of fearlessness. Why did our parents allow such a dangerous expedition? They should not have. I am glad they did. My father might have had a greater inclination to let me take on excessive responsibility and expose myself to danger at this age. After all, he was 15 when he had had to survive on an island on his own. I had managed the farm and climbed Kilimanjaro when I was 16.

Peter recently reminded me that Bill, one of our group, had not been able to go up the last few hundred feet because he felt he was going to fall off the mountain side. When discussing this later with an authority on high altitudes, Peter discovered that this was a very serious symptom, indicating life-threatening levels of mountain sickness. Before hearing this I had always thought that the danger had been exaggerated by boyhood bravado.

I had a glimpse of how bodies might fail to provide these psychological boosts, when a friend David developed polio while visiting Uganda. I remember writing to him as I imagined how horrible it must be for him, and wondering what it would be like for him to have lost the power in his legs. Apparently I was the only one to write. I learned later that David had nevertheless more than proved himself by becoming a disabled East African Safari Rally driver. I cannot imagine anything more daunting.

I left school at 18 planning to go to Cambridge to read agriculture with the avowed intent of returning to manage our farm. I was, however, already wavering a little in my loyalty to this idea, but my parents had already planted trees 'for the grandchildren'. I was thinking vaguely about research in agriculture, which would allow for a way out of this legacy. Between leaving school and setting off to Cambridge I did nine months National Service in the Kenya Regiment, a bruising experience in which I learned how boys were transformed into men who would instantly obey orders to kill. Luckily I never saw anyone to shoot at. We were completely outclassed in the forest by the Kikuyu in the Mau Mau rebellion. Fortunately, they chose not to attack us. An important experience of a different kind was, however, being 'volunteered' to be a medical orderly. I was trained to know the essence of medicine and nursing. I had an interest in how bodies work from my father – in this case animal bodies. He had become an amateur vet on Soysambu where there were vast numbers of cattle and sheep. When any were ill or had died he would be called in to treat them or make a diagnosis on the basis of a post-mortem. I have memories of watching him carry out many post-mortems when I accompanied him on his trips around the farm. I learned what the liver, kidneys, heart, lungs, stomach and gut looked like; what their functions were, which diseases affected each organ and their treatment. He was obviously fascinated by all this, so he made it more interesting for my sister and I. My sister wanted to be a vet. My father's reputation as a vet spread. It was enhanced by the fact that the local qualified vet was nicknamed 'Matador', from his skill at 'killing' bulls. To get the insurance for expensively imported bulls the vet had to be brought in to treat them. This rule was obviously good for importers but bad for insurance companies.

I remember becoming fascinated when the medical orderly training involved watching operations. I watched a gall bladder operation; the operation that my father had had two years before. I also peered into a bladder through a cystoscope. My job was to be the first line of call for troops when they felt ill, and provide first aid. On one occasion a friend of mine became ill after boxing – another training for fighting, which we all had to do. He started having headaches, then vomiting and eventually developed double vision. I knew there was something seriously wrong so went straight to the officers mess. I faced a terrible bawling out for daring to come into their hallowed area, but I stood my ground and insisted on telling them about how ill my friend was. Luckily, they listened as it turned out that he had a brain haemorrhage and had to be flown urgently to London. He survived.

Journey to England

Before setting off for Cambridge I had a holiday on the coast with my parents and then sailed on an Italian liner to Trieste with three friends who were also going to university in Britain. We were planning to spend some time travelling around Europe before arriving in England in September 1956. Sailing north along the Somali coast we enjoyed ourselves, playing a lot of deck tennis. I remember a middle-aged couple watching us and remarking on how fit and athletic we were.

In the Red Sea I started to feel ill; I developed a bad headache and stiff neck. I went to see the ship's Italian doctor who took my temperature. As it was raised he did not ask any questions but gave me quinine – by far the most common cause of high temperature was malaria. We watched the lines of Egyptians standing on the Suez Canal shouting angrily at the ships as they went past. This was just before the Suez crisis and feelings were running high. The headache got worse and, when sitting on my bed, I realized that I could not swing my legs properly and was puzzled by this. I decided to go back to see the doctor. I found that I could hardly walk, swaying from side to side and keeping upright only by leaning against the passage wall. This time I was kept in the ship's sick bay. Quite soon my legs were completely paralysed. The doctor told me that I had polio. I later realized that my polio had been readily diagnosable when still in the Red Sea; as there was a full-blown polio epidemic raging at the time, there was no possible excuse for the failure to diagnose. This level of incompetence was a mixed blessing, however. This was 1956 just before the Suez invasion and if I had been taken off the ship in Port Said or Suez it could have been disastrous.

The medical team was now in a state of panic. I remember vividly how the nurse would come and stand in the doorway of my room looking frightened with feet pointing out ready for flight. She stared at me, glancing occasionally at her watch. I put two and two together and realized that she was monitoring the speed of my respiration. I had seen too many films about iron lungs for polio victims to be unaware of what was happening. I remember being very scared. Nothing was said to me but the question was whether the ship would reach harbour before my breathing gave out. I do not know whether getting a helicopter to take me off was a possibility in those days. I was too ill to think about that. The ship made an emergency landing at Brindisi in south-east Italy and I was carried off the ship on a stretcher with the whole ship watching. I learned later that the captain talked to my friends and selected one to stay with me and told the others to go on to Trieste and then get out of Italy as soon as possible. The one who stayed was Peter – the same Peter of those dangerous ruses. For that I am eternally grateful.

I was left in a corridor in the Brindisi Hospital for many hours. I became very concerned that I was infecting the hordes of people who brushed past the trolley. Eventually they found me a ward. I cannot remember much about the first few days – I was too ill and had a terrible headache and backache. At some point, possibly in a delirious state, I had a fantasy that I had been shot in the back on the deck for running away. Later it occurred to me that the pain in my back coupled with paralysed legs was food for that fantasy. I had, after all, sailed away from national service, which resonated with the image of Admiral Byng being shot on his own quarter-deck for sailing away from the enemy.

Brindisi hospital was a small ill-equipped hospital with only very basic medicine. No one spoke a word of English. Luckily, I had Peter to talk to, but he was only there part of the time and when they carried out any medical procedures he had to leave the room. I soon learned some essential words, such as *dolore* (pain). To establish a diagnosis they did a lumbar puncture, which involved putting a needle into my spinal column and tapping off some spinal fluid. To get me into the right position they put me on my side and then made a rope out of a sheet and put it round my neck and then under my knees and pulled it tight thus bending my back forwards. It was agony because my back was so painful, and my legs had become acutely tender. They did not use any local anaesthetic so the needle was worse agony. When the needle finally reached the spinal fluid and it started pouring out, they did not have a container ready and it all went on the sheet. They had to do it again the next day. That was worse because I knew what to expect.

All my physiological functions below the waist were interrupted for a month or so. This meant that I could not pass urine for a while, so I had to be catheterized every few hours. This was done without any local anaesthetic or lubrication and was very painful. In addition my bowels did not function because I had no abdominal muscles. More disturbing was the loss of potency that follows the acute phase of spinal polio. It lasted many weeks. No one told me, or could tell me, that this would pass. I had a powerful image of a recent newsreel about the polio epidemic in which there had been a girl in a wheelchair being pushed up into an ambulance. There was no doubt about what my fantasies were saying to me.

The most preoccupying issue was what was happening to my legs. I could not move them at all. This was terrifying. To make things worse changes started to occur. Firstly they became excruciatingly tender. It is legendary that polio victims dread even the bed being touched or bumped let alone the limbs being handled. But I did not know this, or that this was due to the muscle dying because the nerves had been killed by the polio virus, or that this tenderness would eventually go. The response of the staff to my immobile legs was, I suppose, instinctual. Beat them into action. Two male nurses came every day to massage my legs. One would stand each side and slap a leg hard and repeatedly. No amount of '*No! No! No!*' made any difference. A more gruesome phenomenon of the muscle dying was the gradual shrinking of the muscle until it disappeared. I watched in morbid fascination as my legs went from exceptionally muscular to Belsen-like skeletons. It is hard to describe the horror of that. It took years to get used to it.

The most welcome event of my stay in Brindisi was provided by a young trainee nurse. She came and stroked my brow muttering, 'Marlon Brando, Marlon Brando'. The most sustaining experience was Peter's warm and caring presence. He rescued my sanity. Recently he told me how difficult it had been for him aged 18 to manage everything. He had to find lodgings and find a way of making himself understood. He was alone and worried for long tracts of time. He also put his own health at risk by staying with me. He told me that it was not until near the end of the stay in Brindisi that he found out that relatives had to bring food in for the patients. The only food I can remember was an absolutely delicious peach that he brought in for me. Obviously the hospital had fed me, but that their food was not memorable. I shall be eternally thankful for Peter's caring and resourcefulness.

During the three and a half weeks in the hospital in Brindisi I hardly slept at all, and constantly watched the ward door. I also got into a routine of glancing at my watch every five minutes. It was not until many years later in studying children's searching behaviour when they are separated from their parents that I understood what that meant. It represented a desperate waiting for my parents to arrive. They never did. It was not until 15 years later that I discovered why. I had accepted the explanation that they were concentrating on getting me back to England and that took all their available resources. I finally asked them what had happened. As soon as they had received the telegram from Peter telling them that I had polio, they went to Government House in Nairobi to open up diplomatic communications with Brindisi and had booked the first available flight to Italy.

At this point, however, my father developed a high temperature and was put into isolation as he was suspected of having polio. My poor mother was in the terrible dilemma of having to decide which male member of the family she should be with. Government House laid on a telephone link with the hospital and for 12 hours she made repeated attempts to speak to someone at the Brindisi hospital but no one could understand English. Eventually she gave up. Luckily my father, who almost certainly did have polio, did not develop symptoms (only a very small proportion do). By the time that my father was better a telegram arrived to say that I did not have polio and had polyneuritis instead. My parents went to see a physician who told them that polyneuritis was a non-infective illness with a good chance of complete recovery. It was at this point that they gave up plans to fly to Italy and instead concentrated on helping to get me transported to London.

If only I had known all this. It would have restored my faith in my parents. When I asked them why they had not told me, they said that they did not want to upset me: 'You had so much to deal with without being burdened by our troubles.' It was a classic case of trying to protect by not talking about something upsetting, but the silence itself becomes the most harmful behaviour of all. I would have much preferred to have been able to feel for their pain and grateful that they tried to come, instead of being left with a 15-year hollow doubt.

The journey to London

In the meantime, Peter was trying hard to get me out of Italy. He went to see the British Consul who was based some 100 miles to the north in Bari. It was a great relief to finally leave Brindisi after what seemed an absolute age. I was put on a sleeper train on the top bunk. I remember stopping at Bari and the British Consul came on board to talk to me. I was so excited that I hauled myself up onto one elbow and chatted away. Peter was appalled at my liveliness; he had painted a picture to the Consul of near death misery. The train then went via Naples to Rome, where I was taken by ambulance to a Convent Hospital. The ambulance journey to the Convent Hospital was strange; lying flat with windows frosted I saw nothing of this great city except for the tops of some grand-looking buildings. Noticing my surroundings was possibly the first sign of my taking an interest in the outside world. In the Convent hospital everything was spick and span and the nuns were very kind; a very different level of medicine.

To fly me to London they had to remove four seats in the plane to make way for the stretcher, and of course Peter had to have a ticket. The expense of my illness was mounting in a frightening way. There were the hospitals' charges too. There were justified reasons for my parents to conserve resources for my impending journey and the subsequent flight home for convalescence. They were not well off and I suppose this helped me to accept their explanation for not coming to England. Maybe. But I was left wondering whether the underlying reason was that my parents were so upset by what had happened to me that they could not face being confronted by it.

Part II: London

We arrived at Heathrow at one o'clock in the morning. I cannot remember the journey to Queen's Square Hospital for Nervous Diseases, but I do remember that the doctor took three hours to examine me. Every muscle's strength, or lack of it, was measured; every detail checked. This was wonderful. At last I had doctors who knew what they were doing. I did not yet know that this was one of the world's greatest neurological hospitals. Experiencing is believing.

Early on in the interview I saw the doctor give the nurse a look that conveyed that all was not right. After the examination was finished he told me that I did have polio, not polyneuritis. This meant that they would have to transform the ward into an isolation ward; Queens Square was not supposed to take infectious patients. I would not be free of infection for another two and a half weeks. I have felt bad over the years about the possibility of having infected other people during my journey and, if I did, had I started an epidemic?

The emphasis now switched to the struggle to get better. I was told about what was happening to me and what to expect in the future. Part of the fear generated in Italy had been due to the unknown. It is better to know what is going to happen, I decided. It was explained to me that the next consequence of the death of muscle would be that the scar-like tissue that was left behind would, as in all scar tissue, start to shrink, thus shortening the muscle, and contracting each joint so that it was permanently bent. Left to their own accord these contractions would lead to me being bent double in a foetal position. So I had to have daily stretching of the muscles, which was very painful. In addition to this, some joints, such as the ankle joint, had to be held at right angles in plaster casts overnight. That was uncomfortable. All this was easier to bear when seen as part of recovering as much as possible. I was told that my muscles would probably regain some strength over a period. Within two years I would know how much muscle I would recover. While the muscles returned I would have to exercise them. There was now a task to take on, a purpose to life.

My physiotherapist was very energetic and challenging, sometimes it seemed too aggressive. But I came to realize that I needed to be shaken out of my state of shock and torpor. I also needed to mobilize my anger. One day she come in and stubbed her toe on the leg of my bed. She hopped around moaning and clutching her toe. I was suddenly cross and irritated that she should make such a fuss when I had such serious problems. I felt very scornful; I could do better than that. It was sometime before I realized that this had been a deliberate and skilful ploy on her part. She regained my respect and I was soon on the way to devoting all my energies to getting more mobile.

I had lost virtually all the muscle in my abdomen and legs. My toes started to show signs of life and by two years I had recovered about 10 per cent of the muscle that I had lost in that area. It does not sound much but I explored many ways of making the best of what I had. I realized later that I had applied the capacity to meet endurance challenges, as well as my athleticism, to the task. In some way this made the loss of athletic ability less horrifying.

My sister Caroline aged 20 moved to London and came to see me every day. That made an enormous difference. I awaited her visits eagerly. She was very sympathetic and held my hand as we talked. I told her about Italy. She was distressed because she had been in Venice on holiday while I had been in Brindisi and would have come south immediately if she had known. Caroline coming to see me and her earnest wish to have been with me in Brindisi helped enormously in healing the wound of being abandoned by my family when I needed them.

By the time I was ready to leave I could sit in a wheelchair and had been wheeled around Queens Square and Russell Square. I remember feeling overwhelmed by the hustle and bustle of people and cars. I was shocked on rounding a corner to be confronted by a shop window that was apparently full of nude women. Everyone seemed to be ignoring these women, which was amazing. Then a man came in and grabbed one of the women, flung her over his shoulder and walked out. I realized that they were plastic mannequins for modelling clothes in the process of being removed from the shop window. I had never seen one before. Nairobi was not like that. I also surprised and puzzled the nurse who was pushing my chair by asking what the notice 'Hovis' meant. I was being introduced to England and its strange ways that all locals took for granted. It was a testimony to how well my parents had brought me up as British that I had been mistaken for a local.

Oxford

After two months I was transferred to the Nuffield Orthopaedic Hospital in Oxford for long-term rehabilitation. One of the nurses escorted me. Although I was lying down in the train most of the way, I sat up for some of it. I was overwhelmed by the beauty of the autumn colours, and by the English countryside, and full of questions about everything. The nurse clearly began to enjoy seeing things afresh through my eyes. We seemed to make good contact. I was excited by the idea of Oxford but when I arrived, I felt suddenly upset and rather frightened. At the hospital I found myself holding on to the nurse's hand and not wanting to let go; I felt abandoned again. I could see that the nurse was concerned and she insisted on coming down to the ward with me. I felt grateful for that. She wrote to me when she got back to London.

Learning to walk again

I spent six months in the Nuffield Orthopaedic Hospital. By the time I left I could walk on crutches. It was very hard and upsetting work. My physiotherapist was more gentle and patient than the one in Queen's Square; each was well suited to her different tasks. She would work with me for long periods each day. In the ward she would continue the stretching of each contracting muscle. It was painful and terribly slow work. She would also get me to exercise the muscles by putting my legs in a sling with pulleys and making me raise and lower weights. This was endurance work.

I also had physiotherapy in the gym where there was a hydrotherapy pool. This was fun. The water was warm and in the water my muscles could do much more as they did not have to work against gravity. It was very encouraging. In the gym there was a walkway, created by two banisters on to which I could hold as I walked towards a full-length mirror. This enabled me to see how I was moving. At first I was very cautious walking on crutches without the banisters and my physiotherapist told me that my fear of falling was hindering progress. I would have to fall to find that it was not a disaster. Here was a challenge. She took my crutches away and I allowed myself to fall. As I recall this I can feel the fear again. Bang. It was all over and apart from a bump on each knee it was nothing. I usually pushed myself down to the gym, which was quite a long way, in a wheel-chair. One day I walked back on crutches without telling anyone I was going to do so. It was a great struggle. News went ahead and when I got back to the ward everyone clapped. Mutual support was so important.

Ward life

My ward had 24 male patients in one long room. Most were long stay with broken legs, bone TB and slipped discs, etc. There was a great deal of banter in the ward. This took the form of teasing and ribald comments about the nurses, and not a little brazen flirting. Someone had given me a little gadget which, if you blew on it, it spun round and read 'I LOVE YOU'. This was much in use to all and sundry. The nurses used to say that they preferred to work on the men's ward because it was much more lively; the women's ward had more talk about how difficult it was, more complaints, and sharing of how upset each was. Which was the more useful technique for coming to terms with disability? Perhaps a mixture would be best.

I started to have a relationship with a nurse. This was great, especially when she was on night duty. She would creep into the ward in the early hours and we would kiss passionately. It was all rather public, but I did not mind that. We were, looking back on it, totally unsuited to each other. She was loud and boisterous and I was quiet and thoughtful, but the ward camaraderie emboldened me – thank goodness. When I left hospital it became obvious that the relationship was not going anywhere but I remain very grateful to her.

I was put in a bed next to a young Oxford undergraduate who had been in his first term at Brasenose when he got polio. This was Jim (J.G.) Farrell, who was to become a Booker prize-winning novelist, though at that time he was in the process of coming to terms with the fact that he would never play rugby again. He had already played for Brasenose 1st XV and had been tipped to get a blue. We used to joke together about the situation. They were sick jokes, which fitted his dry and wry sense of humour. He had been in an iron lung at first but could breathe on his own now. He had lost much of the muscle from the waist up; I had lost almost all muscle from the waist down. We would imagine pooling resources: if we could do that then there would be one completely normal person – great! The other though would be completely useless. On reflection this was probably a metaphor for how each of us felt. The loss of our athletic selves made us feel completely useless, despite having some muscles left. We would often offer each other polo mints with the quip, 'Have another polio.' The empty hole in the middle may have been how we felt.

Sex and its vicissitudes in the face of our disabilities was something that faced both of us. Jokes can hint at impossibly embarrassing issues, while avoiding full awareness of what it is really all about. On the other hand the joke can provide a way of opening up the real issues, but it did not happen that way with us. Perhaps it was too much to expect from two vulnerable young British males. Having read his novel *The Lung*, which was autobiographical in nature, I do know that these issues preoccupied Jim greatly. The front cover picture was of a man hugging a girl who was lying on top of him. With one of his hands he was cutting the strap of her bra with a pair of scissors. His weak hands and arms could not take a bra off. In the book he describes his relationship with a night nurse who came and kissed him in the middle of the night. He commented that the person in the next door bed watched but did not mind. I have no recollection of his kissing a night nurse; he always seemed to be somewhat reserved with girls. I wonder whether he was talking about how he did not mind watching me. A recent biography of Jim Farrell made fascinating reading for me as it gave a picture of the ward life.

There was, of course, another side to ward life. I became fascinated by what was happening around me, such as the development of the nurse/patient relationship and how illnesses affected people. The nurses would talk about other patients and their illnesses to me when they realized I was interested. I learned a great deal. I also learned a bit about death when a patient in a bed opposite died. In the last few days he was curtained off so I was only able to imagine the process. I thought I became aware of his spirit going up to heaven, only to find that he was still alive. The nurses also shared their feelings about him with me. I was beginning to take on the role of listener.

Now that I was in a wheelchair all day I used to go to talk to those who were still bedbound. At first I went to ask if I could draw their portraits. But while I was doing that we would talk. I would ask about the illness and found myself listening to many people's stories and how difficult things had been. I became proficient in portraiture after about 50 drawings. Older men, who were often literally tied to their beds, their legs held by ropes and pulleys, made excellent artist's models with their characters etched out in the lines of their faces. Unfortunately, I gave them all away to the sitters.

I started to go further afield and visited the more serious polio cases who were in respirators. Some of them were totally paralysed, unable to

move anything other than maybe a toe or a finger. Some were in remarkably good spirits despite this. I spent a lot of time with George, aged about
30, who had been in Nigeria when he caught polio. He had been flown
back to England and had been in a respirator ever since. He fell in love
with his occupational therapist and being in a room on his own they were
able to have a serious relationship. They married when he left hospital and
she looked after him until he caught pneumonia and died a few years later
– the fate of most of those serious respiratory cases. It was a terrifying but
deeply moving story; I was inspired by his spirit, her love and their
courage.

I think to some extent I managed my own loss by focusing on those
who were much worse off than myself. Inspired by their solutions, and in
some cases trying to help them to come to terms with the situation, I was
getting my first self-taught lessons in psychotherapy. Perhaps many
psychotherapists are driven to help others who may have similar but more
serious problems. In the process I was working out indirectly how to come
to terms with the polio myself. This was not a bad way of doing it. I came
to see myself as only slightly disabled by comparison, which did not
accord with the reality of my loss. I became proud of the fact that I developed smile wrinkles. Well, why not? But maybe the price is that I am now
having to arrive at a final (hopefully) acceptance of the extent of what
happened to me.

Leaving hospital

On leaving hospital, I went to live in the Colonial and Commonwealth
Club in Oxford. In preparation for this I was taken on a number of outings
to various parts of the city. This was mostly with the occupational therapist, who drove me there, parked and then pushed me around in a wheelchair. I came to appreciate Oxford in early summer, especially along the
banks of the river. I was also taken to various public places by friends,
notably to the Bear Inn at Woodstock. I found it extremely difficult to
manage the walk into the dining room with everyone watching. I was
rather surprised by that. It was the first time I had been seen in my
disabled state by those who did not know me at all and had no reason to
expect to see a disabled person struggling to take a few steps. But I did
manage. A more relaxed outing was a car trip in which I sat in the back
with my nurse girlfriend, got drunk and had a wonderful time.

Jim Farrell was also moving out. He came back very shaken after one
trip to Oxford. He had run for a bus (his legs were normal strength) and
jumped on to the platform as it moved off. As the bus lurched forward he
made to grab hold of the pole, but of course could not even reach out for
it, and so he fell off into the middle of the road. Luckily the car behind just

stopped in time. He said that it was a very scary experience as it was so unexpected, and reminded him of how disabled he was. He looked as if he was normal and everyone treated him as such. The coat he wore hid his Belsen-like shoulders and chest.

Moving in to the club was no fun. I had a first-floor room and knew no one. Either I had to keep in my room most of the time or stay downstairs, rather than struggle to use the stairs on my crutches. I was very lonely. Luckily, I was still going to the hospital for physiotherapy during the week.

Home to Kenya

I now returned to Kenya for a three-month period of convalescence before starting at Cambridge, a year later than planned. Arriving home was painful. My parents met me at the airport and watched me coming slowly down the aircraft steps. I was acutely aware of the impact that this might have on them as they saw the extent of my disability. In a way it also confronted me with that reality. Here I was back where I had been so active not so long ago. My parents managed to put on a good show of just being delighted that I was home. It was later, at home, that I saw my father's look of dismay when I could not move my leg at all; the reality of paralysis came home to him.

I spent some time in Nairobi where my parents now lived. There was little to do in the flat and I longed for the farm. I became depressed and played the few classical records we had over and over again. Beethoven's Fifth Symphony was one, and I am still made sad when I hear it now, with its associations of wartime doom-laden news broadcasts and the petrifying reality of my paralysis. The full extent of what had happened to me was no longer being obscured by the activity and the camaraderie of the hospital. There was nothing to distract me. My mother did her best to cheer me up and told me how proud she was of my courage and determination.

I was given the use of the car and, though I could not drive it immediately, a handbrake was fitted and I started to learn again. I had to retake the driving test. In the meantime I would go for drives with the African driver. We went all over the place. I started to paint some of the wonderful scenery. On one occasion we drove to Nakuru and watched a cricket match at the Rift Valley Sports Club. This was the first cricket match he had watched. He saw this white man run as fast as he could and hurl a stone at a man who only had a stick to defend himself. He exclaimed '*Quayle! Wazungu majinga kabisa!*' (white men really are completely mad!).

My sister came back from London. That was better. She was due to be married in few months to someone she had met while I was in hospital. My sister, my mother and I then went down to the coast for two months. The idea was that it gave me an opportunity to exercise in the warm water of the

Indian Ocean, within the protection of the barrier reef. It was wonderful. Again I found that I was more able-bodied in the water. Snorkling among the coral was magnificent, as usual. I found that if I used a long stick I could anchor myself to the sea bed as well as propel myself along. I could manage so well and stay in the water for so long, and go so far out, that I felt I was back to my old self. My poor mother, quite rightly, felt she had to come with me – just in case. On one occasion she was so exhausted that she almost sank on the last stretch home. I had to return to her to prop her up and help her over the last few yards; I was back to the role of the protector. On one occasion the Italian liner that I had been on when I was taken ill sailed past. It was a strange experience watching it go by.

Then came the news that our farm manager, John, had caught polio and had to be flown down to Nairobi where he was now on a respirator. He had polio as severely as anyone had ever had it. He had no movement in any muscles, other than in a couple of fingers, and was kept alive by the respirator. He conveyed that he wanted to die. The doctors were so dismayed that they asked my father if he would switch the machine off. Of course, he could not do it. My father had been due to join us at the coast, but he felt he had to stay with John, especially as he had no one in Nairobi whom he knew as all his family were in England. Perhaps he wanted to do the bedside looking after that he had wanted to do for me when I was in a similar situation, seriously ill abroad without his family. When we came back to Nairobi I went to see John several times. It was very depressing as he was so suicidal and had no way of achieving it. John was flown back to England and went to the Nuffield Orthopaedic Hospital, the same Oxford hospital I had been in. Eventually he followed the path that my other severely disabled friend George took. He married his physiotherapist and they set up home together. Ten years later he died of pneumonia.

I took the decision that farming was not a sensible career for me. There are disabled farmers, indeed it had been arranged for me to meet one in Oxford. He managed despite being more disabled than I was. But I knew that the frustration of living in the country and not being able to enjoy the wide open spaces would make it a misery for me. I went to see my old art teacher who tried to persuade me to become an artist. He showed me some of his paintings, which stirred my sense of creativity but not enough. My preoccupation was elsewhere. I had become fascinated by the ward life and I had identified with the staff, and wondered about medicine. I told my father about this and, somewhat to my surprise, he was delighted. He told me that he would have done medicine if he had gone to Oxford. I now understood why he was so interested in being an animal doctor.

Cambridge

Before term started I stayed for a few weeks in Hampshire with cousins who generously offered me a home during my studies. I had to buy a car, have it adapted with a hand-operated brake and get myself to Cambridge. It was not easy. I bought a second-hand Ford Popular. I went to collect the car from a garage in London where it had been adapted. The brake had been put on the left side. In Kenya it had been on the right. One of the garage drivers had been employed to go with me to Cambridge. Before we set off he told me how to operate the brake, and then took me to a quiet square. He watched me drive around the square a couple of times, then he directed me back onto the main road and told me to stop next to an Underground station. He told me my driving was fine, got out, said 'Best of luck!' and set off for the station – presumably for a paid day's leave. I was unable to admit that I needed help or that I was scared during the couple of seconds available to call him back.

I looked at the map and decided to have a go. I located the A10 as the road to follow and set off. I got to the first large roundabout where the A10 crosses the North Circular and put my hand out for the brake on the right side – but it was on the left. I found myself sailing out into the traffic, a large Jaguar drove straight at me hooting, but just managed to swerve in time. In my mirror I glimpsed an enraged middle-age man gesticulating wildly at this impudent young man barging his way across. I shot out onto the A10 with a flying start not having slowed down at all for the round-about. How I negotiated Royston I shall never know. All I can remember was getting hopelessly lost and eventually arriving in Cambridge from the wrong direction. I eventually came to a halt on Queens Road when I recognised Kings College Chapel on the other side of the river. I asked the first person who came along how to get to Clare Memorial Court. My luck was turning. He was going there himself, it was just round the corner, and I had someone to help me find my room, unpack the car, and take my things to my room. I had been worrying how I was going to do all these things with the two sticks and no hands free to carry anything.

Now the real trials began. I discovered that all meals were served in Clare Old Court, which was about a third of a mile away across the river Cam. So off I hobbled to have dinner. The first three weeks were a bit of a blur in my memory. Finding how to get to the lecture theatres was one thing; driving there was another. I discovered the hierarchy on Cambridge roads reversed all my previous experience. Pedestrians came first, stepping out onto the road without looking, knowing that the swarms of bicycles would divide and pass either side. Cars came last – if at all; especially first thing in the morning five minutes after lectures were supposed to have started. This was definitely not how it was done in Kenya. I found myself stuck at a major junction not being able to move until someone in the car behind got out and enquired if I needed a push, assuming I had broken down. Eventually I devised a method of edging out slowly across the avalanche of swarming bicycles, shouting apologies all the way. That seemed to work.

After three weeks I was half-asleep with exhaustion. But I would not give up. I went to everything, even the things that were eminently missable, such as chapel. I had been brought up on daily chapel at a British colonial boarding school so I knew exactly when to stand up and so on. I noticed my tutor watching me carefully as I struggled to get myself upright. He approached me afterwards. He had already explored alternative lodgings for me where I could be fed without the constant marathons to the dining room. I immediately accepted. I think he knew from my demeanour that I had had to try it out till I nearly collapsed before I could accept any sort of compromise.

My first teaching experience was to walk (hobble) into a huge room with 70 dead people lying naked on slabs. There was a strong smell of formaldehyde. Dissecting may not have been as foreign to me as to some, as I had done so many animal post-mortems but on people it was initially chillingly weird. The speed with which everyone became familiar in the presence of the dead was unnatural. Soon we were leaning on our elbows on 'George' or 'Mabel' as we chatted. The lively familiarity was with other young students, I watched several romances flourish within a day or two, while dead people became objects that could be cut up with scalpels. The meaning of all this, developing different attitudes towards ill or dead people from personal relationships, did not dawn on me until much later. We became familiar with death and by the end of the first week we were well on our way to becoming the typical, boisterous, irresponsible, fun loving, young, medical students.

For me a more significant problem with dissecting was that it was very tiring. I had to lean over at the same time to use both hands while I dissected out a nerve or a piece of muscle or eyeball. As I had no trunk muscles I had to prop myself up with my elbows, which restricted what I could do with my hands. It was a relentless process because we had to keep to a group schedule. Every week or so each student had to pass a viva during which we had to demonstrate that we knew the names of every dissected nerve, muscle, or bone, as well as describe the spatial relationship between each of them. We had to identify them on the cadaver and show that we had exposed each part correctly. I would return to my rooms exhausted knowing that I had to pour over my anatomy books that night. We dissected in pairs. My partner was Carol, a very bright and studious girl from New Hall, who went on to get a first. She was very kind and we got on well together. This helped as she did much of the dissecting, but it had to be done meticulously. As I write I am particularly aware of how my anatomy dissecting was only made possible by her. One of the great gifts of having a disability is receiving so much kindness that is generously given. Writing this makes me want to thank everyone with a hug.

There were other aspects of the medical training that posed massive physical challenges for me. Many of the courses, such as physiology and biochemistry, had practicals which involved manipulating materials or chemicals on laboratory worktops. I laughingly called it cookery. I became more and more tired. Eventually it became clear that I would need to have some concessions. Luckily the course lent itself to this. Most students, but not everyone, did a specialist subject for their third year. I was however, quite legitimately, allowed to complete the Natural Science Tripos over three years, which enabled me to space the practicals out and made the course just possible. It also cleared enough space to start enjoying the intellectual stimulus of Cambridge. That was precious.

The strength in my legs slowly increased until the end of the first year (i.e. two years after the illness). Even though I had still lost 90 per cent of the muscle of my trunk and legs, those muscles that I did have were well distributed. For instance my quadriceps on the right side is missing but the left has about 15 per cent recovery. The calf on the left side is missing, with 20 per cent remaining on the right. The result of this was that I am able to use one leg to go one step at a time up stairs using my one quadriceps, and stand on tiptoe with the functioning right calf muscle. I was also always apparently ahead of the recovery schedule. The doctors had told me origi-nally that I might have to use a wheel chair but that proved to be too pessimistic. The physiotherapist in Oxford had ordered a set of callipers for me. By the time they arrived I did not need them as one of my quadri-ceps had recovered sufficiently to climb some stairs. I started on crutches and progressed to walking sticks. By the second year at Cambridge, I was impatient to take the next step. I flung both my walking sticks into the bushes in Clare Fellows' Garden. Although good for morale this was a step too far for practical good sense. I kept falling down.

Probably one of my most stupid decisions, but also one of the best, was to insist on my right to have a room in Clare Old Court in my last year. It was on the first floor. Once I fell down the spiral staircase and pulled a ligament in my knee. That was no joke as I was confined to my room for six weeks. The only lavatory and bathroom were across the quad on a cobblestone path, and then downstairs underneath the chapel. Once I fell twice while walking on the cobblestones across the quadrangle. My knees were very sore. At least the college dining room was on the other side of the quad, not the river. It was an inspired choice, however, because it put me where I could be uplifted by the wonderful views and some sublime music. My rooms were huge, bitterly cold, and had no mod cons except a coldwater tap on the landing. They were on the corner of the court next to King's College Chapel; one of the world's most beautiful buildings, with some of the world's greatest choral music. I could hear the choir many times during the day and evening.

From the window in one direction I could see the whole length of the chapel and in the other right down to the river Cam. At times I would stand at the window of my room watching the girls go by. When there was work to be done I would take my books down to the banks of the Cam and watch the girls go by in punts, the books unread. When things were difficult I might go and sit in the chapel, sometimes for hours, gazing at the infinitely delicate fan vaulting floating high above me, or watch the sun light up the brilliant colours of the medieval stained glass windows; a fiery ball of light, forever changing colour as it passed from pane to pane. I would feel myself merge with its beauty and space, perhaps in a way similar to how I had disappeared into the grandeur of the Rift Valley. This was a spiritual experience.

Religion played a role in my emotional recovery. It was hard to know when it started – perhaps in Italy. I found that I could create a sense of God's presence especially when very alone in the middle of the night. I felt a profound relief – at the presence of a concerned parent at last? I bought religious books about the spiritual significance of pain. That was a mystery that had been thrust upon me; surely it must have a higher meaning. The crucifix turned pain into a transforming experience. It was not until I was in my last year that I lost my faith. One of my American friends asked me how I could think that the Anglican church had the one true link to God when there were thousands of religions all claiming the same thing. Nevertheless religion has had an important place in my coming to terms with experiences that could otherwise have left me alienated and abandoned in despair. I could feel somehow that I had been on a purposeful and ultimately redeeming pilgrimage. I can now see that the suffering may have transformed my being in a way that was towards growth and creativity, even if not to godliness.

My parents came to England while I was at Cambridge. I showed them the sights, including, of course, King's Chapel. My father told me later that he had had a profound religious experience there. Sadly, he was trying to make religious links with me just about the time that I was relinquishing mine. Perhaps the two events are linked. The real presence of my father was what I had wanted, not an imagined substitute. As I write this I wonder what might have happened if I had known about his suspected polio from the beginning. I imagine that I would then have had an image of a father wanting desperately to come to me but who was also struck down. Maybe we could have shared a desperate sense of enforced separation, not a sense of abandonment on my part, and probably guilt and regret on his.

As is common with many university students I had to come to terms with the fact that my mind was in the middle range of ability at Cambridge, rather than the high range, as at school. Nevertheless, I started to enjoy the level of debate and searching for answers to questions that abounded. I found the tutoring system very enriching. We usually went in twos to the tutor on a weekly basis. Here we could be exposed to the thinking processes of some of the brightest people in their field. I was lucky to have Professor Wilmer who was a major pioneer in colour vision. My fellow student later became a don at Clare himself and made his own contribution. I was witness to the joining of two creative minds. They had to slow the tutorial down to make it comprehensible to me, but it was very exciting. I cannot remember any of the content, but I can remember how absolutely everything could be questioned. Hypotheses could be conjured up that stood accepted ideas on their head. I was also interested in wider issues such as philosophy and went to some lectures given by the appropriately named Professor Wisdom. It was fascinating. He would philosophize with himself in front of hundreds of students. He would start by reflecting aloud on some issue, apparently lost in deep thought, and would then ask a question. Then he would race off to the other end of the lecturer's bench to answer it, which would lead to a further question that would have to be answered from the other end, and so on. It was great theatre, vividly illustrating the process of philosophical debate.

In the last year I became the President of the East Africa society. It was amazing that key people would accept an invitation from a mere boy of 20 to come to talk in public in Cambridge. The title 'President' does not suggest a boy, I suppose, and Africa and its colonies were centre stage of international politics at that time. I think we managed to arrange an interesting programme. I wrote to colonial governors, writers on African issues, senior politicians and many others. We managed to persuade Michael Blundell, who was pioneering multiracial solutions at the time, to come. Most importantly and memorably, we invited Tom Mboya. He was one of the most inspiring Kenyan politicians of his era, and strongly tipped to be a future leader. I was very impressed with him at every level: as a person; his charisma and his political ideas. There were many hundreds at the talk. I cannot remember being anxious introducing him and chairing the meeting; Cambridge self-confidence was beginning to brush off on me. Tragically Mboya was murdered not many years later. It is dangerous to be too promising.

Friends provided my psychological lifeblood. On the first or second day I met Tony at an organic chemistry tutorial and we have been close friends ever since. He was a scholar and was extraordinarily helpful over the time at Cambridge in a multitude of ways, including helping me to revise before exams. We had a number of holidays together, including staying at his home, and one memorable trip to Scotland. For my last long vac in the summer of 1960 I toured Europe with old school friends, Mark and John. Mark was the person with whom I had had the lion hunt and he was now farming in Rhodesia, while John was also at Cambridge but was reading agriculture, the subject that I had originally planned to study. The tour started in Paris; Mark had been lent a friend's flat. To our dismay we discovered that it was on the seventh floor and there was no lift. I had to be carried up piggy-back. In the evening, I stayed in the flat while John and Mark went to a night club. They came back with two Danish girls. I was very jealous, which unfortunately I turned into disapproval. Later, it became more difficult as the two of them had more in common with each other than with me. I was more interested in cultural things and my artist self was beginning to predominate over the farmer self. Sexuality, however, was somehow caught up in it all. My Kenya self still saw farmers as more virile than artists.

By the time we got to Florence it was vital that I went my own way. Mark and John wanted to go to the 1960 Olympic Games in Rome. That was the last thing I wanted to do, so I told them to go ahead. I was anxious about coping on my own but I also knew that I needed to establish that I could manage my life. We had been staying at the youth hostel (Mussolini's old summer home), or rather its grounds, as all the rooms were full. I had made friends with an English teacher in the next tent who knew Florence well. I would offer him lifts in the car: he would show me round and manage anything that I could not deal with. It worked very well. I had brought a wheelchair with me, and discovered that I could see the sights far better using it. I spent days in the Uffizzi, and explored most of the great sites of Florence with the aid of my new-found friend, who was a very knowledgeable guide. I sat for two days in the Academia drawing the amazing Michelangelo sculptures. I chose two to draw, firstly David; a perfectly muscled man. Then I drew the Pieta, in which Christ is being supported by two women. It was a powerful experience to draw it, feeling for his flaccid legs, flopping as if they were paralysed, and marvelling at his massive strong arms. I was using drawing to explore my loss of athleticism, now only to be found in my arms. I do not think I was aware of doing so until I had finished. I had portrayed myself before and after polio. Interestingly this is also the focus of this writing. Earlier in hospital I had drawn a charcoal picture of the crucifixion when in a state of high

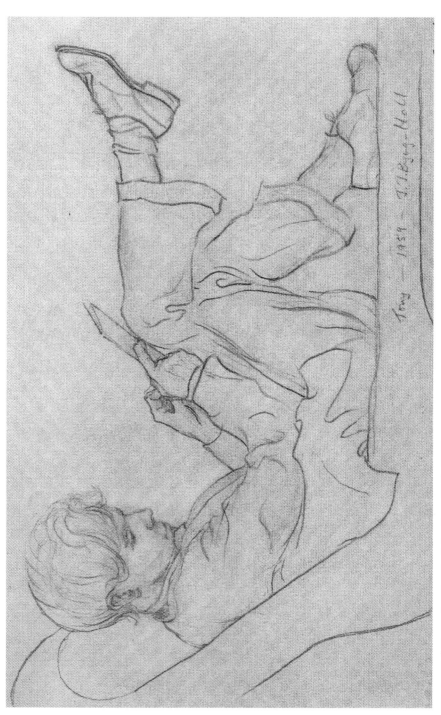

Figure 1.4 Tony: drawing by John Byng-Hall, 1959.

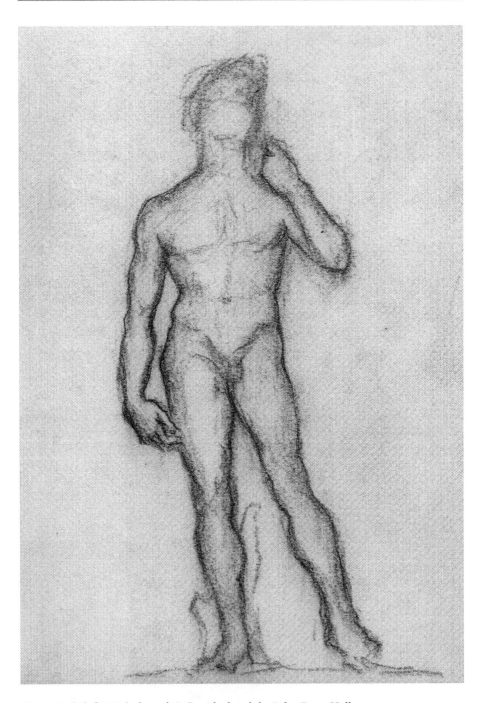

Figure 1.5 (left) Michelangelo's David: sketch by John Byng-Hall.

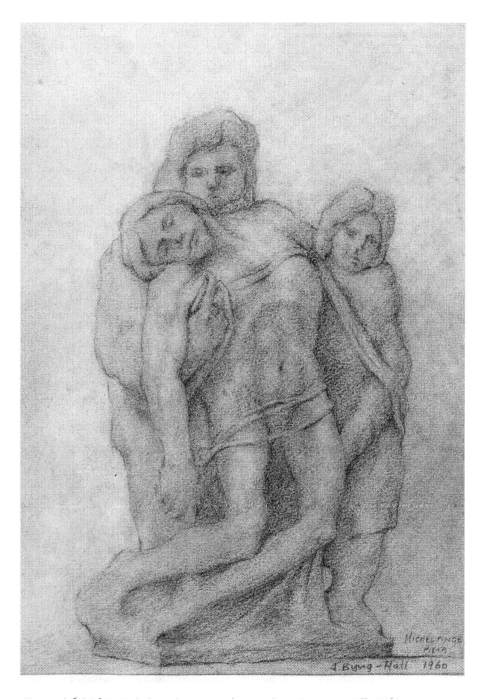

Figure 1.6 (right) Michelangelo's Pieta: drawing by John Byng-Hall, 1960.

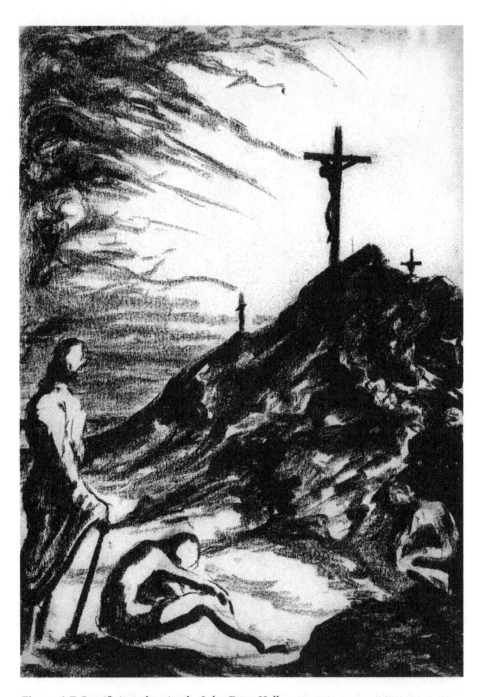

Figure 1.7 Crucifixion: drawing by John Byng-Hall.

emotional tension and at high speed. I had drawn three men in the foreground; one sitting looking down at the ground in despair, and the second standing with a stick looking up at the cross, and the third merging into the hillside below the crosses. I was exploring the process of emerging from depression and learning to stand and walk through the inspiration and security of being in the vicinity of Christ who could conquer pain. As I write this I am not sure whether I had seen the significance of this drawing so clearly before. Now, with my knowledge of attachment theory, I see this as a way of conjuring up an attachment figure in a threatening situation.

Jim Farrell and I kept in touch, on and off. He had a good friend, Roger, in Clare who became our link person. He was a mature student on a scholarship from America, interested in publishing and editor of *Granta* at the time. One day Roger came up to me very excited and told me that Jim had written a novel that would undoubtedly be published. He gave me a copy of the first half to read. The story, as I remember it, was a rattling good yarn about young people's lives. A few days later Roger came to see me again looking gloomy. He had read the second half and had serious doubts that it would ever be published. The hero, without warning, suddenly developed polio and was in an iron lung. It was shocking, and portrayed a life suddenly turned upside down. Our mutual friend thought that it was too shocking and disconnected to be readable. He was probably right. The book portrayed a similar incomprehensible disjunction between health and disability with which I struggle now. Jim rewrote the novel and called it *The Lung*. This second version was less disjointed as he started the story, now featuring an older man, in the early hours of the illness, retrospectively painting something of the picture of his life before polio. To me the first version carried far greater impact. The descriptions of being in an iron lung, however, were the same in both versions and remain very powerful. *The Lung* never sold well. Jim's struggle with writing about his past was one of the stimuli that encouraged me to write this memoir. I wanted it as it had happened.

Finals were followed by a great outburst of activities and parties and May Balls. I was at a loose end. Suddenly I was on my own, not fully part of what was going on. All my friends were looking to the next stage in their lives. Male camaraderie, fostered by the all-male colleges, was rapidly being replaced by girl friends and going off to work around the world. I had a place at University College Hospital in London to do my three years of clinical training. I was very worried about how I would cope. The training did not start until the autumn and this was June. I stayed on in Cambridge, and became depressed: a piece of mourning that I had put off for four years. I started to draw and paint Clare, as a way of holding on to Cambridge, I suppose. I now sense that it was rather like holding on to the hand of the London nurse when I transferred to Oxford. For me Clare was essentially feminine, not only because of its name but also the images of Old Court's soft beauty. Fittingly, it became the first college to accept women that was to lead to the end of the dreadful inequality of one woman to every seven men, which was so damaging to each sex.

First, I did a pastel drawing of the doorway to the chapel in one corner of Old Court, which was very beautiful, and carried many important memories. It was also a way of recording a mirror image of the entrance to the staircase to my rooms in the opposite side of the court. The other picture was an oil painting of Clare Old Court and Clare Bridge painted from the Fellows Garden across the river, where my sticks lay somewhere in the bushes. I did not finish it, although it was promising. Perhaps the half finished state was symbolic? I still had some grieving left over. I have it in mind to finish the picture now. Perhaps this writing will help.

London: University College Hospital

Arriving at UCH was daunting. The Medical School and Hospital buildings in Gower Street were large and rambling. This time I made no mistake about where I lived. I had a room right next to the medical school dining room. The queue for meals snaked past my bedroom door. This was distracting but it allowed me to be much more sociable by dint of allowing my friends a place to sit while waiting for the canteen to open. I had a great deal of walking or driving to get from clinic to clinic. At some point I acquired a shooting stick to walk round the wards; I would prop myself on it for the interminable bedside discussions. More tiring was when I had to assist at operations and stand for hours at a time. I forced myself to volunteer for case presentations because I knew that I had to manage those if I was ever to get through the medical training. I was frightened of the possible public humiliation through the interrogation, the way that some consultants, mostly surgeons, attempted to make us think while under stress, and in the process establishing their own pre-eminence. I also worried about managing the physical examinations of patients. Somehow I found a way, but it was far from easy.

As I tell the story I do not have a sense of burden surrounding this period of my training. I think I was wafted into the busy routines and the major crises that hospitalization created for the patients. I remember spending much longer talking to my patients than other medical students did. I was picking up from where I had left off my own hospital experience. This is what I came into medicine to do – become involved with my patients in the drama of illness in a ward setting. UCH was very advanced in its approach to psychological issues. There were regular ward rounds in which psychiatrists discussed how the illnesses and the ward setting influenced the patient's experiences. We were also told to read John Bowlby's 1953 book, which had come out of his study of the distressing effects of separating children from their parents during the war. This had involved studying hospitalized children. Not surprisingly, this rang loud bells for me. As well as this all medical students took on one patient for psychotherapy under close supervision.

About two-thirds of the way through our clinical training we were all pondering which branch of medicine to specialise in. Not surprisingly, I had wanted to be an orthopaedic surgeon but by now it was clear that I could not manage the carpentry involved. I could manage rheumatology, which works with similar medical problems but, disturbingly, I had also come to realize that I found illness and its routine medical care very boring. The contemplation of endless clinics with hundreds of arthritic patients coming for adjustment of their drugs was soul destroying. I became depressed when I faced the possibility that medicine had been a huge mistake, especially considering the mammoth struggle involved to get this far. The depression eased when I realized that what did interest me was people's reactions to illness, not the illness itself. At about this time I elected to have a student placement at a rehabilitation unit. They had made the interesting discovery that using group methods to motivate those recovering from broken limbs reduced the time it took to return to work when compared with standard ward physiotherapy. It became clear to me that I could have a greater influence on recovery by knowing how to manage the emotional issues than mastering medical methods, confirming my own experiences as a patient, though I was not fully aware of the connection at that time. I resolved to do some psychiatric training after qualifying. From there it was natural to discover that the human psyche was the most interesting thing on earth, and I decided to work in child psychiatry in keeping with preventative principles. Later, when I told my father that I wanted to do psychiatry, he was appalled. Did I want to look after 'nutters'? But true to character he quickly regained his composure and steadfastly supported me.

A year before I qualified as a doctor I married Sue. It is impossible to overestimate the importance to me of my marriage, three sons, and granddaughter. This is where my life flows. But I must keep to my pledge not to include them in this writing. Suffice it to say that I am weeping with gratitude and loving warmth as I write this.

House jobs

The highest hurdle of all still lay ahead: to qualify I had to do house jobs. At that time there was a tradition that a house job was for six months –

nothing more, nothing less. You were on duty for six months, 24 hours a day, seven days a week. I recognized that this was impossible for me, so I searched the journals for the few jobs that had some time off. The first was as a house physician in the geriatric unit at UCH, which had the luxury of every other night off. The most enlivening memory comes from a patient of 108, at that time the oldest person in Britain. Everyone loved her. She used to say her prayers 'God help Amy, Grace, Edith, etc.', clearly her childhood friends of a century ago. One story was about her daughter, aged 85, who, coming to visit, asked directions of the hospital porter to find her mother's ward. He rang the resident psychiatrist: 'We've got a confused old lady here, doc.' This job was manageable and I even found the time to sit and draw her. This time I kept it rather than giving it to her. She could not see.

I was dangerously tired for the following two six-month jobs. The worse one was a paediatric job at Addenbrookes Hospital in Cambridge in which the last ward round was held at 1 a.m. Once or twice a week I would be up most of the night with a newly born, seriously ill baby, but nevertheless would have to start the morning ward round as usual at 9 a.m. I had a half day off mid-week, and alternate weekends (which meant that I stopped work at 7 p.m. on the Wednesday and Saturday) and went home and slept. I was no use at all to our eldest son who was now one year old. In addition I was the houseman for ophthalmology, which entailed admitting twenty patients a week for operations on their eyes – and going to the morgue to remove corneas for transplants. Just outlining this schedule appals me. I get a cold dread in my stomach, as I recall it. I did not knowingly kill any children, but if I did not do so it was only by good luck. The most painful job was telling some parents about the death of their son whom I had admitted the previous evening. I learned nothing about paediatrics because as soon as I opened a book I fell asleep. The present large academic paediatric department simply cannot believe that one consultant (internationally known and also editor of a famous paediatric journal), a part-time consultant, one registrar and one part-time disabled houseman comprised the team that looked after the sickest children in a large part of East Anglia.

Another important experience was being the surgical houseman for an ENT ward. Fifteen to twenty small children would have their tonsils and adenoids cut out in an afternoon, some by me. Later that evening the ward was hell with children weeping and crying with pain – and calling for their mothers. Parents were only allowed to visit twice a week for a brief period, 'because it upset them and made them cry starting off bleeding'. I gave a copy of John Bowlby's *Child Care and the Growth of Love* to the ward sister, who thought it 'rubbish'. She was a very nice and level-headed person, and I

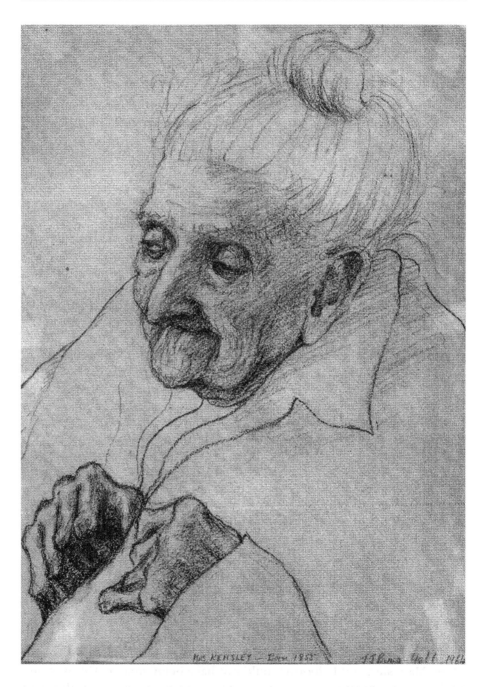

Figure 1.8 Mrs Kemsley, born 1855: drawing by John Byng-Hall, 1964.

was confronted by human beings' capacity to eventually become selectively deaf to children's crying, especially from the distress of separation.

Adult psychiatry training

I spent 1965–68 as a registrar at Fulbourn Hospital. It was an amazingly advanced mental hospital run on therapeutic community lines. I had specifically applied for a job in a therapeutic community because of my experience of the rehabilitation unit at UCH where the patients supported and encouraged each other. There were no locked wards at Fulbourn. My most remarkable experience was working as the psychiatrist for the disturbed ward while the consultant was away on a six months' sabbatical. It was reminiscent of my running the farm, aged 16, in my father's absence. The patients were extremely disturbed, the most troubled and troubling in East Anglia, who could not be contained anywhere else. All the decision-making was done in daily community meetings. It was remarkable to see how mature and knowledgeable the patients were, especially about what would be best for each other, and of course they took ideas from each other more readily than from staff. My role was often to take heed of suggestions for changes in drugs. For instance, 'Doc, I think that Jane [someone who became extremely violent in the relapses in her psychotic illness] needs a slight increase in her medication.' They could tell. I learned how profound the influence of social context could be on people's behaviour, without going over to some of the anti-psychiatry ideas that were circulating at that time which assumed that all madness was socially induced. Without medication the doors would have been locked.

I recently reread an unpublished article that I wrote in 1968 in which I said, 'The major therapeutic event which occurs in a patient's stay may be that he finds he can change his role e.g. after spending many years as the rejected scapegoat in his family, he finds himself as the ward chairman.' The one criticism that I had of the ward was that little work was done with the patients' families to enable patients to leave and live at home. From Fulbourn I went weekly to a two-year course in psychotherapy for registrars at the Tavistock Clinic. This and the therapeutic community set me firmly on the journey towards psychotherapy. I decided that I needed a more thorough training and had been advised that the best way of getting a job at the Tavistock Clinic was to go first to the Maudsley.

The contrast between The Villa, which was the locked disturbed ward at the Maudsley, and Fulbourn could not have been greater. This was one of the world's great psychiatric teaching hospitals; the idea that they had anything to learn from junior doctors from provincial hospitals was unthinkable. Not able to comment I became an observer, particularly of hospital rituals. My first experience was of the Professor's Conference, with about 60 people present. The new recruits were ushered to the back. At the front sat other professors and dignitaries. The registrar, soon to be me, gave a very fluent and apparently anxiety-free presentation to the assembled company. The patient was brought in, seated in front of the audience and then quizzed by senior staff. My knowledge of group process made me acutely aware of how this man might be feeling about this public exposure. The main preoccupation of the professionals was intellectual competition. They seemed oblivious to the emotional impact on the patient or on the registrar, who was also quizzed in a way designed to catch her out. The powerful lesson for the junior staff was: 'The intellect unbiased by feelings is what matters in staff; the feelings of patients are phenomena to be examined.'

The lie was out when I heard the registrar being congratulated afterwards on how calm she'd appeared. The information required was apparently scripted in great detail in an admission document, so if it was followed carefully you would be safe. Just to make sure, you also needed to spend many hours asking every conceivable question and exploring every avenue surrounding your case. In that way you could manage one of the most frightening social situations possible to devise, and show courage by not showing fear. My family had trained me well for that. The staff had all been trained at the Maudsley in this way and, though they must have known the fear at some level, they presumably considered it good for trainees. After all they had learned not to be anxious, so felt free of emotional bias. The basic format of the Professor's Conference was reproduced at every level in the hospital, including at each ward round. It was in the bones of the place.

When it came to my turn to present I went in on the attack. I talked to the new Professor about changing the ritual. I had some videotape of a boy of six with a low IQ who could read anything – Latin, English verse or German etc. – in a phonetic way, a skill he may have learned by sitting for most of his life in front of TV adverts, where the product's name was both spoken and written. I argued that we could not get him to demonstrate this phenomenon in the context of the conference but the video showed it very well. He agreed, but was hesitant about removing the staff's right to question the boy. As I left the Maudsley soon after this I never knew whether this started a new tradition.

Child psychiatry

I worked for six months as the registrar to the Maudsley's Children's Ward, an impressive place for 30 disturbed children. In the day it was buzzing with high-powered professionals but, as I discovered, at night there were

only three night staff and bedlam reigned. This was never talked about and
the ward was rarely visited by senior staff at night. My family experience of
seeing beyond the public façade that camouflaged what was really going
on, especially at night, had sensitized me to such situations. Nevertheless,
I also learned a great deal at the Maudsley and met many very nice,
thoughtful and capable people. While there I read the first of Bowlby's
trilogy about attachment theory, when it first came out in 1969. I was now
keen to make the move on to the Tavistock Clinic as a Senior Registrar
towards the end of that year.

I worked half time in a new adolescent unit in St Albans. Work started
with the whole family at the point of deciding about admission. Here was
the missing side of the therapeutic community at Fulbourn. Those in
parental authority were given as much, or more, responsibility as the adult
patients in Fulbourn. Understandably, the only reason for offering
inpatient as opposed to outpatient treatment was whether or not the
adolescent could be coped with at home. This decision could only be
made by parents or social workers for those in care. The decision to
discharge could also only be made by parents, so regular family meetings
were arranged to review whether the family could now cope with their
adolescent at home, usually after weekend visits. There were no guidelines, as far as we knew, for this form of family work in the literature. We
explored what happened in families by putting into words what we saw
happening within the family – in other words we became narrators to the
family's interactions. In this way we learned about family process and
family dynamics, and how to support parents to make their decisions
about admission and discharge. Salvador Minuchin spent a year's sabbatical at the Tavistock in 1972 and described one of the aims of structural
family therapy as restoring authority to parents. Although these ideas did
not influence the early form of family work starting in 1969, it gave same
validity to our approach.

I became interested in a form of family belief that was common in many
of these families, who idealized themselves and scapegoated the adolescent. They might, for instance, believe that they were very honest, unlike
their son, though it would become clear in family meetings that this was
far from the case. In 1973 I conceptualized this consensus belief as representing a family myth. I had learned in my own family about this form of
consensus belief that the family has about itself that contradicts what is
actually going on. My family believed that it was 'very close' but there were
many ways in which this was not so (especially in not sharing worries),
and we emigrated to different continents to achieve autonomy.

The other half of the senior registrar job was in the Adolescent
Department at the Tavistock. The department meetings were a mirror

image of the Maudsley. The greatest value was given to being sensitive to one's own feelings evoked by patients, in other words the counter transference. This was valued as a source of information about what was happening in the relationship with the patient. In these meetings there was a similar degree of competition in displaying the greatest degree of insightfulness as there had been in the intellectual competition at the Maudsley. Perhaps all institutions that see themselves as centres of excellence are likely to use a ritual that encapsulates the underlying beliefs.

The social injunction to trainees at the Tavistock at that time was that they must have their own psychoanalysis and if possible become psychoanalysts in order to become successful therapists. To go into analysis required even greater courage for a stiff upper-lip, proper Englishman (and Kenyan to boot) than braving the Maudsley den, or facing a charging elephant! Good heavens! Do you mean lying down on a couch and sharing every intimate and taboo thought as it comes into my mind with a strange lady, five times a week for years! You must be joking – and *surely* not dirty Freudian phantasies about her too – NO! To justify this terrifying step I had to see it as a necessary part of my training though I still needed a push to get into analysis. This came in the assessment interview for the psychoanalytic training with Michael Balint. Balint was one of the world's experts on why people became doctors. He took me apart. I gathered afterwards that he had a reputation for making people change in one interview. His last comment did the trick. He said that he still did not know why I had become a doctor. I took this to mean that I should not have become a doctor, and I was devastated; crying on and off for three days when alone. Not until writing this did I realize that Balint was referring to the very issue with which I am now struggling – the incongruity of my transformation from farmer to doctor.

In the event my analysis turned out to be the most valuable corrective experience to my family's taboo on sharing any worries. But it was far more than that. The relief of being able to tell someone my unabridged polio story was immense. To be heard and sensitively understood without my having to worry about the effect on the listener was a great relief. I had been just as constrained as the rest of my family by the idea of not upsetting people with the truth. I had to visit this scenario soon after starting when my analyst was off sick for two weeks. Had my story been too much for her? It was a painful start, but useful, as it went to the core of the problem immediately. It turned out that her illness was not one that I could have possibly induced.

The discovery that so many things could be understood using so many avenues was very enriching. I found out that my analyst had been analysed by Marion Milner, who had written a book about using art as a form of self-exploration. Bringing my pictures to her became an important and enlightening part of the process. I could express the full horror of the polio in picture form. I discovered that she was not full of crazy Freudian ideology but was down to earth. (I had deliberately chosen an analyst from the independent group as I could not tolerate the idea of dogma.) It was a relief to find that she did not interpret my snake memories as phallic symbols. She pointed out that laughter was an important part of human nature, giving me licence to use my humour. Towards the end of my analysis she told me that she thought that being sent to boarding school at the age of seven had been more damaging psychologically than the polio. I think this is right. It shattered my absolute trust in my parents, and set up a distancing form of self-sufficiency, which influenced many other things, including how I handled the polio. One of the most precious gifts of analysis is discovering how to take care of yourself in an intimate way that embraces all aspects of yourself, the murky as well as the loving side. This helps one to care about one's clients in a similar way. The self-exploration involved in this writing is clearly an extension of that tradition.

As I became more focused on family therapy, I would discuss the families with whom I worked and found my analyst's thoughts very helpful. I could start to try to disentangle the feelings and impulses to act in family therapy sessions coming from my own family experiences, from those being evoked by my client families – and to see how they mutually influenced each other. My analyst was helpful in supporting my decision not to complete my psychoanalytic training, despite completing most of the seminars. I was no longer wanting to be an analyst, and continuing would have involved spending 24 hours a week training, while working a full-time contract as a consultant at the Tavistock Clinic. I also had a family with three young sons – and was disabled. One of my greatest regrets was the amount of time and energy taken away from my family in order to manage my job. My analyst helped me to make a common-sense decision.

I was open to any good ideas wherever they came from. I explored the theories proposed by family therapists, mostly from the USA, which usually involved a distancing from psychoanalytic ideas. In the early days most of the pioneer family therapists had been psychoanalysts, but they seldom acknowledged that their own analysis had played an important part in the skill and speed with which they tuned in to what was going on in families. We were witness to this particular skill as we invited many of the world's senior family therapists to London in the mid-1970s and 1980s, as a way of informing ourselves and spreading the family therapy gospel to others. At the same time as joining the exciting process of pioneering new ideas in family therapy, I was building on what I had learned 'back home' in the analytic world. I now realize that this is similar to what the Kenya pioneers had done with farming.

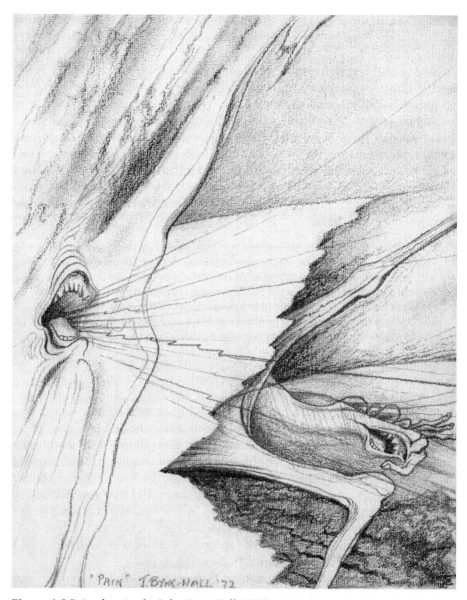

Figure 1.9 Pain: drawing by John Byng-Hall, 1972.

Where did my story take me?

Through these reminiscences I discovered a number of things. I can see that I am the same person after the polio as before. This now feels obvious, although I could not readily put the two images within the same frame a few months ago. How did this come about? I had written a 'writing diary' recording my experiences of writing as I went along, which provides some clues.

Recalling many of the more difficult episodes from my past was painful, and at times I was reluctant to go on. It seems that I had been avoiding thinking about some of my past to prevent the distress of recall. I was surprised at how upset I was when recalling episodes in my earlier childhood, such as the terrible shock of going to school at seven years old, and being terrified during the Mau Mau rebellion. Perhaps I had focused most of my energy over the years on either thinking about, or actively avoiding thinking about, aspects of the polio which then distracted me from working out earlier traumas? The polio, however, was even more difficult. To quote from my diary:

> I felt very relaxed when writing about the early part of the trip (on the boat to England) but as I started on the process of getting ill it became much more difficult, even more so than the Mau Mau. At times I would feel so upset and repelled by what I was writing that I would seriously think about giving up. At the worst point (when describing my time in Brindisi) I decided to do something different and read a paper I had been sent to review. Soon after that, I found that I could return to writing my story without wanting to avoid the pain.

Regulating the intensity by focusing on something that needed my full attention, such as a review, may have helped.

I felt much more relaxed after I had reached the point where I was recovering from the polio. Energy flooded back and I felt creative in a whole number of ways. However, as I wrote about the struggle to cope in Cambridge, I felt weighed down and faced the quandary of waiting or proceeding – which strategy would work better? I tried to pause but it did not work as I had no energy to do anything else. After a couple of hours I decided to read what I had already written. After all I had reached adulthood in England in my story. Reading my story seemed to help me to de-role. I could step back from reliving the raw experience and reflect on it again. I then felt motivated to write the rest. Enthusiasm returned, and I continued my story up to becoming a family therapist.

I was then able to read it afresh, using the story told to 'a stranger' as a story to myself. I could trace the transition between active health and disablement; childhood and manhood; Kenya and England; country and city; farmer and family therapist. This enabled me to see how there was continuity between past and present. It was now possible to envisage that I might have become a doctor and family therapist even if I had not had polio. There were many antecedents: my father's childhood interest in medicine and how he later channelled this ambition into being an amateur vet and my mother's early experience of VAD nursing and later as

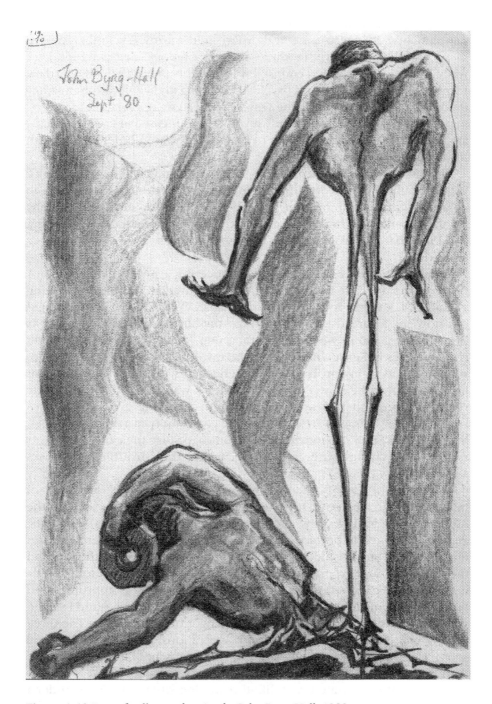

Figure 1.10 Fear of collapse: drawing by John Byng-Hall, 1980.

a nurse/doctor to many people on the farm. There was also my own sampling of medicine as a medical orderly in the army. Psychotherapy was in my blood, listening to 'mother's knee psychology' that emerged later when I wasa self-appointed counsellor to patients in hospital in Oxford. As I wrote about my clinical and psychiatry training and exploration of family therapy it became clearer to me why I had become interested in families, in particular how to decode family mythology expressed in family stories. I am keen to enable the unspoken to be talked about in order to deal with the fantasy that it is unspeakable.

The other central theme in my work has been attachment and distance within families. This is no surprise: my family had this tendency to go to different continents in order to leave home, and I was subjected to many painful separations during my early life. All this makes more sense now, and I feel that I know better my own capacity to see my particular ghosts around me.

Finally, I am aware that it was the pioneering aspect of family therapy that fired me up. Here I was carrying on my Kenya family tradition of being a pioneer. I could be loyal to my family legacy even if it was not farming. I can now see a thread running through my life of self-sufficiency that is provided by a group working together. Our family had to cope with all contingencies in Kenya. In hospital I was involved in the self-help aspect of ward life, and in my professional life engaged with the energy of client groups to solve their own problems. When I was a medical student, the rehabilitation unit that speeded up recovery using group processes sparked my enthusiasm. The therapeutic community in Fulbourn carried this on, while family therapy enables families to solve their own problems rather than having a therapist treat each of their troubled members separately.

This piece of reminiscence has helped me to look at my own 'state of mind' about attachments. It is this state of mind that is revealed by the Adult Attachment Interview about memories of childhood attachments. Perhaps the most important experience that this writing offered was to find that by its end I could go through the story of my past, all the joys and the deep pain, and experience all the appropriate feelings as I told it. This is the essence of coherent narrative in which the affect is appropriate to the episode being described. As I typed it out the first time I found I stalled with the pain of certain memories; a harbinger of incoherence. The three stalling points were all associated with separations; going to school aged seven; the Mau Mau uprising when I was away at school more of the time than at home, and finally contracting polio on leaving home. The latter two were both associated with life-threatening situations. No wonder I was interested in attachment theory. I have become more aware of the various ways in which I have struggled to make sense of what happens to me in traumatic situations, through art and talking about difficulties.

Attachment researchers are interested in 'earned security' in which those who have had adverse life experiences that might have been expected to lead to insecurity are, nevertheless, able to tell a coherent story about it, with all its anger and pain, and are likely to have securely attached children. In this piece of writing I am confronted with evidence of a trauma that was still not fully resolved. Would I have been rated as U (or unresolved mourning) on the Adult Attachment Interview, soon after my illness, or until my analysis, or even until recently? For an unresolved classification the narrative has to break down at the point of describing the unresolved loss. I remember telling the whole Brindisi story to a cousin who was a contemporary of my mother's when I was in hospital in Oxford. It was felt deeply in the telling and, as she reported, in the listening too. Perhaps this indicates that I could tell a coherent enough story soon after the polio. But I do remember thinking that I had lost some of my memory, so perhaps it was not the whole story that was told. I have had the huge advantage of a stable and what felt like a secure early childhood, and then psychoanalysis. Nevertheless, I feel I have tasted something of that struggle to 'earn' a sense of security, and it leaves me in awe of how those without these advantages manage to retain their sanity.

One way of explaining my inability fully to place the image of my athletic self next to the disabled self was because it was too painful a reminder of the loss. This had hindered the completion of mourning of my athletic good health. Colin Murray Parkes explains how mourning is the process of giving up the original assumptions about the future with the person or function that has been lost. This involves a long process of repeatedly bringing an image of the lost person or function into mind, followed by the awful realization that he, she or it has gone forever. This goes on until the reality of what has happened is fully accepted and a different set of realistic assumptions about the possible future is put in their place. I probably had not quite completed that process, and had put my athletic self out of mind. Some of the assumptions about who I would have become were still there, though, which would be incompatible with how I am now. Hence my difficulty in seeing my muscular self side by side with my paralysed self. Perhaps reminiscing is likely to throw up some uncompleted mourning. If so it provides an opportunity to finally come to terms with what happened.

John Bowlby (1988) and Mary Main (1985) suggested that having incompatible internal working models for the same situation can lead to incoherent narrative. I had two incompatible internal working models of potent manhood. My Kenya model of manhood implied courage in action.

Inaction was cowardly. I can remember lying in bed in hospital in Oxford watching the Russian invasion of Hungary on television and thinking that at least I now had a reason why I could not go to war. The spontaneous relief was followed immediately by an intense shame at having had the thought. The 'semi-retired English family therapist' on the other hand considered that the courage to pause and think, despite pressure to act immediately, was the mark of creative manhood. These two images of myself were difficult to reconcile. Attributing the transformation to a maturing process did not seem a good enough explanation. That, I assumed, would have led to a completely different mature person. I feel that this writing did involve the final mourning of my athletic self, so that the same person made the transition from past to present, and I could accept the paralysed state, which made me more rather than less of a man.

The power of the story came from the experience of reliving the 'Kilamanjaro climbing man', and onwards, in a continuous stumbling journey, into the experience of a reflective city therapist sitting in his office. One of those stumbles was loosing potency and athleticism simultaneously at the onset of polio, a confirmation of my childhood assumption that physical prowess was a sign of potent manhood. Recovering my balance took two steps, first finding after a month that this link was not so, and the next by having a family of my own. That changed everything. This final linking has released me to face the second wave of loss, as my muscles lose more of their strength in the post-polio syndrome. Facing that is painful but it does not threaten me as a man. Consequently I am free to make realistic plans to adjust my life so that I can continue to enjoy it, instead of struggling up what feels like an ever steeper hill, too scared to notice what was happening to me. This experience has hopefully also made me more sensitive to what disablement might symbolise for those families that I see who have a disabled member.

How do family and couple therapists work on their own inner families and make sense of it? Almost all forms of individual therapy require that the trainee undergoes an experience of the same form of therapy for themselves. Very few family and marital training schemes ask for this of their trainees. How could you justify bringing relatives in to therapy just for gaining a professional qualification, unless it becomes clear that it is necessary? Many other ways of exploring the inner family are used instead. As I discovered individual therapy can be very helpful. Family trees can be drawn or recreated in family sculpts, and many other family-like group experiences provided. Perhaps what I have described here might provide another way of increasing the coherence of one's narrative about family life.

I now feel much more at ease with myself and can recommend reminiscing in this particular way. But be prepared to make enough time and space available. It took me two months of writing, for several hours, most days – but then my story had to cover 62 years. It may be harrowing at times, but I found ways of managing without withdrawing. Those moments of anguish or despair now feel to have been the most valuable for me. For others it may be different. Moments of forgiveness of one's parents, and oneself for that matter, may be more profound.

I have now realized that one of the reasons for writing this memoir was to bear witness to the experience of disability and the necessary adjustments to it, which most people do not have to experience, but need to understand about disabled people. Before writing this I had not seen myself as disabled, but as a person who had a disability in mobility that only needs addressing when it interfered with my normal life. This seems to me to have been an appropriate attitude to take, despite the tendency to overstretch myself by ignoring the extent of my disability. Now, with an increasing lack of mobility I see myself as someone who needs to focus my attention on disability in order to adapt my life to it. Perhaps this is what we all have to do when aging. Semi-retired I now have great joy in painting. I have finally accepted that I need an electric wheelchair and with it I can now reach beautiful parts of the country – and paint.

Chapter 2
The first family systemic training course

ROSEMARY WHIFFEN AND JOHN BYNG-HALL
IN CONVERSATION

John Byng-Hall worked at the Tavistock Clinic from 1969 to 1997. He was joined by Rosemary Whiffen in 1972, and they became Co-Chairs of the Family Therapy Programme in 1974 until Rosemary's retirement almost 20 years later. This is a conversation between them about their work together, the clinic which provided a setting for their collaboration, and about the outside influences and connections that contributed so much. The Tavistock Clinic is a National Health Service clinic that provides psychotherapy services in north London. It is also the premier postgraduate teaching centre in psychotherapy in the UK. John Byng-Hall and Rosemary Whiffen worked in the Department for Children and Families.

RW: We both agree that when we arrived at the Tavistock Clinic there was a seedbed for something different to emerge at the clinic, despite all its established ways of working. What do you think contributed to this seedbed and who do you think was influential there?

JBH: John Bowlby wrote one of the first papers on family therapy in 1949, which he used to unblock impasses in individual work (Bowlby, 1949). When John Bell heard about this work he started working exclusively with whole families in the USA. In this way Bowlby influenced the development of family therapy in the United States and was a consistent supporter of family therapy (Bell, 1951; Byng-Hall, 1991).

   There were other influences, for instance, Ronnie Laing who worked for a while at the Tavistock and created a worldwide culture of thinking about how parents could contribute to their children's emotional disturbance. I think he got some things wrong. Much of his work was with young people and he didn't see their contribution to what happens but rather saw the parents as the cause of the youngster's problems. He seemed to be siding with the adolescent against the parents, so the idea of mutual influence was lost. But still, as a forward thinker, he was remarkable and we shouldn't forget that.

RW: There were a number of others at the Tavistock who were interested in families at the Tavistock in the fifties and sixties.

JBH: Yes. We should also remember that Freda Martin and Jane Knight, supported by John Bowlby, wrote a paper in 1962 recommending that all therapy should start with a family meeting. This set up a tradition within the whole department.

RW: We really did inherit a fertile field. Freda Martin also played a crucial role in the organization of the department.

JBH: One of her most important political influences was that she became Chair of the Department of Children and Parents at the same time as being Chair of the Family Therapy group. This provided the sort of political clout that enabled family therapists to flourish, even if what they were saying at times went counter to the central beliefs of psychoanalysis.

RW: Yes, we could experiment and explore and plant the seeds of new ideas and methods without them being weeded out and trampled upon.

JBH: But it was also interesting that it was through conflict that a lot of things changed. For instance, it was almost impossible for family therapy to thrive while there was an interdisciplinary intake and treatment team assessing each case, which created competition between each member of the team. For instance, the child psychotherapists would, naturally, argue hotly for individual work for every child. This meant that very few families were able to move smoothly into family work. The Department as a whole decided that they were ready for a change, so when Freda became Chair in 1972 she reorganized the department. Instead of everyone being allocated to a multidisciplinary team, groups were organized around interests and approaches. This meant, for instance, that people who were interested in working with families, whichever discipline they came from, would work together. In this way the shared approach allowed each group to develop its own thinking and expertise, and helped us to move out of the conflict between different approaches.

RW: Freda also established a new move away from the necessity of having the psychiatrist in every team hold clinical responsibility on every case. You were part of that, I believe.

JBH: Yes – I was the newest consultant and under Freda's leadership we discussed with the Medical Defence Union how to allow clinic responsibility to be delegated to other disciplines. This also allowed family therapists to be involved as soon as the family walked in the door, without the child having to see a psychiatrist first. This, I think, influenced practice in the rest of the country too.

RW: Yes, I remember well. Without that arrangement family therapy could never have taken off. Before we got to the Tavistock we were both reaching out to work with families. What had already influenced you to do this?

JBH: I suppose I have to go back to when I was a medical student in 1961 at University College Hospital, where every student was supervised in psychotherapy.

RW: As part of your medical training?

JBH: Yes. It was very progressive and a very formative experience. I was working with a young woman who had asthma and lifelong problems. I got nowhere and I came to realize that one of the reasons was because of her difficult family experiences. At the same time I was reading a book on the history of medicine. The book described how when developing ways to tackle an illness, medicine usually started with diagnosis, then went on to treatment and finally to prevention. It struck me that the treatment of disturbed adults was very difficult, so the most valuable thing would be to start with prevention and work with families. I had this idea in the early sixties and I had no idea that family therapy existed, although later, when I did my psychiatric training in Cambridge, I found out that John Howells was working with families in Ipswich and I went to see him work with a family. I then heard about Robin Skynner, who was a family therapist, so I knew it existed.

      I should perhaps add one very important influence. When I was a medical student, I had been told to read John Bowlby's book *Child Care and the Growth of Love* (Bowlby, 1953). I was so impressed by it. There was no jargon, I could understand it and it made such good sense. One of the reasons I wanted to work at the Tavistock was because Bowlby was there.

      But you also searched for ways to work with families before you came to the Tavistock.

RW: Oh definitely. I think it is interesting that Bowlby's *Child Care and the Growth of Love* also had a great influence on me. When I was training as a medical social worker it was a seminal book that we were all told to read. Later, when I was a medical social worker at St Mary's Hospital and later still when I was a senior tutor at the Institute of Medical Social Work, I was also greatly influenced by two psychiatrists who were also psychoanalysts: Fortunato Castillo, who consulted with our department on seminars for the staff, and Anthony Storr, who lectured the students at the Institute on Human Growth and Development. Both of them not only put great stress on early life influences but also emphasized the importance of later life experiences and ongoing family relationships.

In 1969 when the Institute of Medical Social Work was disbanded and the training moved into the universities, I decided to look into the whole issue of family therapy. I made enquiries around the UK but did not find any real opportunities at that time, so I decided to take up a job I had been offered in a Mobile Crisis Unit situated on the Lower East Side of Manhattan. This was part of a most exciting new project with unique opportunities for trying out systemic ideas. The unit was part of a neighbourhood hospital that was divided into interdisciplinary units where the family was seen as the patient. The aim was to provide across the board health and mental health care to family units. The mental health care was headed by Edgar Auerswald, a systemic family therapist and theorist. The Mobile Crisis Unit was separate from the hospital and based in the community to allow for flexibility. It was directed by another psychiatrist and family therapist, Emery Hetrick.

The Unit served a multi-ethnic, poverty-stricken area. It consisted of an interdisciplinary team which included professionals and para-professionals, who came from the local community and who had been specially trained in the new approaches. They were drawn from the different ethnic groups: Puerto Rican, Black, Jewish, Italian and Chinese among others. It was a great learning opportunity to experience the application of new theory and approaches. I was also able to attend seminars, workshops and conferences run by established family therapy institutes and to meet and get to know a number of leading family therapists.

From there I came to the Tavistock in 1972 when Mary Barker was Senior Tutor of the Social Work discipline. She knew of my experience in the United States and was interested in the whole concept of systemic family therapy.

JBH: During those same years, from 1969 to 1972, I was also gathering my first experience of working with families. I had a very interesting job, half time in the Adolescent Department, pioneering psychoanalytic ideas about families, and the other half of the job working with families in the Adolescent Unit at Hill End, St Albans, where we used a family approach with adolescents, who were admitted to the mental hospital.

RW: Peter Bruggen set it up, didn't he?

JBH: Yes. We first tried three times a week psychoanalytic psychotherapy
      for those adolescents. That was very challenging! I remember one
      session when the adolescent pinned me down and dialled 999
      behind my back. The first I knew of this was when the police and the
      fire engines arrived! We found that groups worked better. We also
      evolved a way of working with families. We asked ourselves why an
      adolescent should be admitted to an Adolescent Psychiatric Unit in
      the first place. We considered it very important not to label children
      as being mad, as they might then adopt this identity, possibly for the
      rest of their lives. The only way we could make sense of having in-
      patient treatment, rather than out-patient treatment, was when their
      parents, or whoever had parental authority over them, couldn't
      cope with them in the community. This then became the reason for
      admission, not because of a psychiatric illness. This led to working
      with families and how to help them to manage once again (Byng-
      Hall and Bruggen, 1974).

RW: What about the other half of your job?

JBH: At that time I was one of the people who set up the Family Therapy
      Workshop in the Adolescent Department. There was also a research
      group that we started in 1971. The four members of the research
      team studied family therapy sessions using videotape recordings.
      We were exploring how object relations theory could be adapted to
      understanding family systems.

RW: Were you using the one-way mirror at that time as well?

JBH: Yes. That's another thing about the Tavistock. The use of one-
      way mirrors had been going for some time, but video was new
      and initially frowned upon for clinical work. Video arrived in 1971
      and I was involved in setting this up with Jimmy and Joyce
      Robertson, who made the world-famous films showing the impact
      on children of being separated from their parents on admission to
      hospital.

RW: It was Bowlby and the Robertsons who were responsible for the
      change in policy in hospitals, which led to parents being allowed to
      stay with their children in hospital.

JBH: Yes, that was one of the biggest direct influences the Tavistock has
      had on family life. So the tradition of film was already part of the
      Tavistock ethos and its successor, video, provided a vital tool for
      family therapy. We could review what we had done and observe the
      impact. Families are so complex and things happen so quickly!
      Reviewing videotape became a very important part of my thinking
      about my work.

RW: It did for me too. In fact for all of us, I think. So we have looked at our original professional lives and at practical experience with families. Our own ongoing 'training' in family therapy was piecemeal, but nonetheless rich and varied.

JBH: Yes. We started to learn together when I got a job in the Children and Parents Department and the two of us joined Freda in setting up the workshop for all the staff of the Family Therapy Programme. It provided the context in which we could continue learning.

RW: Very soon we started the first training course in family therapy and our trainees joined us in those morning workshops. We explored ideas, read books and articles, discussed them and analysed videotapes. We also used experiential exercises and techniques like family sculpting, role-play and sharing our family trees. Although these workshops became part of the training course it wasn't a training session for them only.

JBH: No. We were all learning together and it was very exciting.

RW: It certainly was.

JBH: We also integrated ideas from the outside world, both from the literature and by making contact with family therapists from abroad. It was a very rich mix.

RW: Yes, and at this time we began to have connections with American colleagues, like Sal Minuchin who spent a sabbatical in 1972 at the Tavistock and wrote *Families and Family Therapy* (Minuchin, 1974) during that time. That was an important experience although I don't think we were ready for him, but it sowed some seeds.

JBH: You had the idea of bringing in the Ackerman Institute in New York, one of the leading family therapy institutes where you had contacts, and to invite them to participate in two joint conferences. We saw families and presented tapes ourselves to the conference members, alongside Don Bloch and the other Ackerman staff members. Although the difference in experience and skill was very evident at that time, I think we established an important principle that we could be participants in the development of those new ideas and not just recipients of outsiders' wisdom.

RW: Yes. We also ran three residential conferences in Cambridge with US colleagues from various institutes. All these conferences had a great impact on the development of family therapy in the UK, I believe. Besides these overseas influences, the group of UK colleagues which Robin Skynner brought together in 1972 to set up a family therapy course under the aegis of the Institute of Group Analysis was also of great importance to us. He invited family therapists from leading organizations in London, the Maudsley, Great Ormond Street and the Tavistock, to name a few. Working together on this project, the staff of the course became colleagues of enduring importance to us. Eventually this group became founder members of the Association for Family Therapy, a national institution, and later the Institute of Family Therapy, a London-based training institute.

JBH: Right. Following the first Ackerman/Tavistock conference, one of the significant although sad events for us was that Freda Martin decided to go back to Canada. At that point the important decision was made that the two of us should co-chair the Family Therapy Programme, rather than one or the other.

RW: That was a very important decision for me but why was it from your point of view?

JBH: I think I needed a partner and needed your expertise because you had a lot of ideas from your time in the States. Also, it seemed to me that it made more sense to have shared male–female leadership in the group. It seemed important to 'model' a family, in which men and women carry shared authority. Anyway, it certainly turned out to be very important for me because of the energy and inspiration you gave to the whole process. I think I was probably the reflective person and you were the initiator and got things going.

RW: It meant a lot to me too. I enjoyed our sparking ideas off each other and I have always greatly valued your way of coming to a decision. You never 'toss off' an opinion but always take great trouble in coming to a considered position.

JBH: This is fascinating because I always remember you saying, 'we have really got to think this thing through'.

RW: Really? But perhaps there was also a complementarity between us in the way we saw the implications of some of the innovations we were making, but you certainly had the edge on vision and originality of ideas. I also enjoyed the shared responsibility of a co-chair arrange-ment, not only for the male–female partnership, but also for the stimulation provided by having the two disciplines of psychiatry and social work heading up the programme. This was also very impor-tant when we had to relate to the outside world.

JBH: It certainly was.

RW: Mind you, we sound as though we had an easy road all the way but we have to remember that it was not always plain sailing. In view of the political situation in the clinic we had to learn by trial and error. To begin with, I think we were so enthusiastic about our new ideas that we encouraged people with other views and orientations to come and see what we were doing. Our enthusiasm was not always shared and the results were not encouraging! We then became very unobtrusive and made as little noise as possible. Predictably we then became the focus of suspicion. Finally we learnt to be open about our ideas but to present them as different, without an undercurrent of judgement about what was right or wrong, better or best.

JBH: We have to hand it to the clinic. We ended up practicing and teaching in a way that broke all the rules, but they supported us nevertheless. I think one of the most important decisions that we made when we became co-chair was to focus our training on those applicants who had the potential ability to become teachers themselves. We developed a part of the training that was aimed at teaching how to teach, based on courses that trainees set up in their own communities while training with us. As ours was the first family therapy training in the UK, it was the only way we could set up something which would have a wider impact beyond the training organization. It proved to be a strategy that created the widest spread of family therapy expertise, as our trainees developed their own approaches, and many went on to set up their own teaching groups.

RW: Yes. I think that was a far-reaching decision.

JBH: It also led to us staging the first International Forum for Family Therapy Trainers in 1979. That was a remarkable event as a high percentage of the world's leading family therapists came, and it had never been done before. I always think of that occasion as the moment that we came of age in the world of family therapy. Our book about supervision came out of it (Whiffen and Byng-Hall, 1982).

RW: What about later developments for you?

JBH: Well, I became increasingly interested in research issues. Family therapy theorists had developed a number of concepts to explain how disturbed families functioned, thus providing a rationale for techniques used to help families. But there was no theory about families that had been adequately validated by research, and so could not be ignored, on which these theoretical constructs could be based. One of the results was that new ideas were constantly displacing previous wisdoms. The field became fashion conscious; the latest ideas were praised and we flocked to hear the latest prophets, while last year's became old hat.

RW: Do you think this was something to do with family therapy's pioneering ethos?

JBH: Yes. Like the original pioneers each of us just had to share the latest idea that we had discovered. Very exciting in a way – and very competitive! This process abated later with the rise in the interest in the philosophy of power (White and Epston, 1990), which helped us to realize that the theories that we thought up, as well as our own cultural and family assumptions, could be imposed on families, when we should be listening to their stories. This realization was very helpful, but in the end families wisely want a therapist who has ideas about what is likely to be going on, so that appropriate action can be taken. Research can be in the position to provide the most probable explanations of what is happening, as well as seeing whether particular approaches do produce change.

RW: What research issues interested you?

JBH: I had been very intrigued by Bowlby's ideas about attachment. I was lucky enough to collaborate with him in various ways during his very long and fruitful retirement. What was fascinating was to hear him become increasingly excited as an ever-increasing number of research projects confirmed his theory. Here then was a theory increasingly validated by research that was central to family life, which had been shown to be clinically relevant as insecure attachments are associated with more problems than secure attachments. What is more it suggested various techniques which, when I tried them, seemed to be helpful. Most important of all, attachment theory makes sense and everyone, including our clients, can understand it. Attachment research tells a good coherent story, and it is fascinating.

RW: What aspects of attachment have interested you?

JBH: I have been thinking about concepts that put attachment into a systemic framework. In particular I have been elaborating the concept of the family as a secure base (Byng-Hall, 1995a) in which the family is experienced as providing emotional support when needed and so contributing to the sense of security for all its members.

I have also been interested in what light attachment research throws on narrative. In 1985 Mary Main and her colleagues (Main, Kaplan and Cassidy, 1985) published some research on narrative. They found that parents of securely attached children could tell a more coherent story about their attachments during their own childhoods than parents of insecure children. There are various forms of incoherence each of which fits a particular form of insecurity, but one common feature is that the incoherence reveals a particular difficulty in dealing with past memories; either blotting out memories of painful episodes in relationships, or being preoccupied with memories of how unfair their childhood was, or suddenly losing flow when recalling unresolved losses, for instance talking as if a dead parent was still alive. Insecure children are more likely to develop problems than secure children. It seems that the capacity to be readily in touch with the experience of your own past pain and joys in relationships is helpful for children because the parent can quickly empathize with the child by recalling what it felt like when they were children. This lies behind the capacity to respond sensitively and appropriately to their children's distress.

RW: You had your own ideas about narrative before this research, and before it became fashionable in family therapy, didn't you?

JBH: Yes. In the 1970s I had been interested in family belief systems embodied in family myths (Byng-Hall, 1973), stories (Byng-Hall, 1979), and legends (Byng-Hall, 1982a), and later in family scripts, which are what families do about their beliefs (Byng-Hall, 1998). I found that I could relate much of this to the new attachment research. I worked for ten years on the concept of family scripts (Byng-Hall, 1985). Attachment is only one part of family life, albeit an important part. The concept of family scripts, however, is about how all aspects of family life are enacted, so it provides a good conceptual framework for integrating attachment issues into family therapy as a whole. The result was my book *Rewriting Family Scripts* (Byng-Hall, 1995b). Since then I have been thinking about how to help families provide a more secure base by helping them to tell a more coherent story about their attachments (Byng-Hall, 1997, 1999a), which is an example of research leading to ways of helping families. I have also been involved in presenting a family and marital perspective to those interested in attachment (Byng-Hall, 1999b), which hopefully will contribute to a dialogue between attachment researchers and family therapists.

RW: How do you see your life and work when you look back?

JBH: Well, on the one hand I would like to be starting now! Probably the most fascinating story about families is beginning to be told. On the other hand, I see this situation as an outcome, in part, of all of our early work and I feel very privileged to have started when I did, and to have worked with such talented colleagues at a pioneering stage.

Chapter 3
Letting go of attachments

David Campbell

Introduction

I first met John in 1973. I was a newly qualified clinical psychologist who had just arrived from the USA to work in the health service. Camden Social Services Department had recently opened a Reception and Assessment Centre for children taken into their care, and they appointed John, a child psychiatrist, and myself, a clinical psychologist, to carry out assessments and staff support. These were joint appointments, which meant that we worked part-time at the Child and Family Department at the Tavistock Clinic. John had begun his career at the Hill End Adolescent Unit, where he and Peter Bruggen pioneered a family approach for adolescents who were admitted to an in-patient unit (Bruggen, Byng-Hall and Pitt-Aikens, 1971). When he took the post in Camden, he was determined to carry on with this work in the new setting. Having recently completed my own training, I was very keen to try my hand at educational and personality assessments, employing a full range of projective tests such as the Rorschach and the Children's Apperception Test (CAT).

During our first year together, I saw John take the child and staff members back to the family home for 'family meetings'; I saw him comforting families recently torn apart and confronting families who could not manage adolescent separation; I saw him dealing with violence and abuse and mental illness; I saw him drinking many cups of tea and climbing endless flights of stairs when the lifts in blocks of flats had broken down. Above all, I admired his courage. Gradually, I and most of the staff, were converted by the power of this approach to heal family rifts or, in some cases, to make it possible for children to leave dangerous family situations. The Centre established the practice of two types of meetings: the professional meeting, attended by workers such as social worker,

72

teacher, general practitioner and family members when appropriate, whose focus was to discuss the decision-making process facing all involved in the case; and the family meeting, usually attended by John or myself plus the worker from the Assessment Centre and various family members. These latter meetings generally took place in the family home and I remember many of them as stormy and poignant, because the issues of losing a family member and the intrusion of the local authority into family life had to be faced.

In the early 1970s the prevailing model of family therapy was structural, and its emphasis on parental authority and appropriate generational boundaries was extremely helpful in our family work. But John lead the centre staff toward a more eclectic model which incorporated a variety of family therapy techniques from the field and interwove his own thera-peutic preoccupations. For example, John was very skilful at reaching the painful hurt feelings which inevitably lay beneath the angry blaming attacks. I recall him using the phrase 'moving from blame to pain' when he described this work. He was also planting the seeds of his lifelong interest in family scripts. Every family session included a family tree to explore the experiences of loss and separation over generations, and sculpting techniques were frequently employed to unblock difficult feelings in the family. Because we were presented with a child at some stage of care proceedings, we also needed a conceptual model which enabled us to connect the 'identified child' to the wider network of family relationships. John was instrumental in developing the idea of the child as the 'distance regulator' between the parents for the types of families we were seeing in Camden, and a number of papers were written on this subject during this period.

Meanwhile, at the Tavistock, John and our social worker colleague Rosemary Whiffen established the first family therapy training in Britain in 1975. The staff group of five or six worked with a similar number of trainees, in an atmosphere of 'learning together'. For example, every Thursday morning staff and trainees gathered for an experiential workshop at which we would do sculpting and simulations of our therapy work. The training course had extended visits from Sal Minuchin and Marianne Walters from the USA, and was heavily influenced by their struc-tural family therapy techniques. However, as the training course devel-oped and each staff member began to clarify their own approach to therapy and live supervision, differences, inevitably, emerged.

The Milan team presented themselves to the family therapy field with an article in the journal, *Family Process* (Selvini Palazzoli et al., 1974) and their seminal book, *Paradox and Counterparadox* (Selvini Palazzoli et al., 1978). I found, for example, that their interviewing style of working from a systemic hypothesis and asking connecting or circular questions enabled me to build a clearer picture of the family as an interacting system. Simultaneously, it allowed me to create the optimal therapeutic distance between myself and the family, so that I could be empathic without being overwhelmed (Campbell, Draper and Crutchley, 1991). The Milan approach offered an alternative method and validated the need for different styles among the different personalities in the family therapy team. John and Rosemary had been the pioneers of our service, but I needed to get out from under their shadow, if I was going to develop my own ideas.

A similarly minded colleague, Ros Draper, and I ran a live supervision group for two years which included three very enthusiastic trainees, Peter Lang, Martin Little and Claire Fidler. We all decided we would run the group along the principles outlined in *Paradox and Counterparadox* (Selvini Palazzoli et al., 1978), and very much learned the method together. Some years later we were joined by another colleague, Caroline Lindsey, to establish a two-year family therapy qualifying course which was specifically based on the Tavistock version of the Milan approach. For several years the two family therapy courses ran side by side in the same department, as the best way we could find to develop the thinking and practice of the different models. At times this was very uncomfortable as, it seemed to me, John would have liked to have us working more closely with the family therapy model he was developing, but it was also inevitable that our differences would be expressed in different trainings.

In the meantime, John was articulating the theoretical model, attachment theory, which underpinned his lifelong interest in the replication of family scripts through history. He was involved in several research projects which identified different patterns of adult attachment behaviour in parents with current patterns of behaviour among their children. The research, teaching and tireless, dedicated clinical work with families, ultimately came together in the writing of his book, *Rewriting Family Scripts* (Byng-Hall, 1995b).

As is the case with most neophytes, we tried to perfect the model which we observed from afar and make it our own by developing our Milan therapy techniques and by applying the Milan model to public service settings in the UK (Campbell and Draper, 1985). Once the euphoria of using a new proven method began to recede, we looked at the differences between the Milan method and the 'British' version. For example, we discovered that many of our client families did not fit the profile of the closely knit, passionate, extended Italian family, but were rather cooler and more cut off from extended family ties. This meant we had to develop more hypotheses about distant or separated families. We found that many of our client families had become entangled with helping professionals and, in order to be effective, we had to think of these relationships as essential parts of the family system.

The core concepts

But there were also specific ideas within the Milan approach which attracted us and set us and the method apart from other family therapy that was going on at the time. The most important of these was undoubtedly the concept of neutrality. This concept, more than any other, distinguished this new approach from the 'schools' of the original founders of the family therapy field, who tended to be active, persuasive, charismatic and largely male. Neutrality enabled less active, less charismatic therapists to be powerful and effective and, in my view, ushered in a new generation of family therapists. It is a concept which has been used in many ways, from the aim of seeing every point of view as valid and worthy of understanding to the suggestion that a therapist should remain value-free and unconcerned about whether there is change or not. I think there are serious flaws within this latter position and I am adopting, here, the former definition of neutrality.

Neutrality gives the therapist a platform from which to take a broader, more systemic perspective of family interaction. We are all too familiar with the feeling of being dragged into one way of seeing a family and losing the ability to generate new ideas; from this platform, and with the benefit of a more systemic perspective, the therapist can begin to make statements or ask questions that explore the connections among the different parts of the system.

The technique known, perhaps inaccurately, as circular questioning has become firmly associated with the Milan approach, as the basis of the therapy interview. At the heart of this technique was the conviction that therapists were trying to help family members see themselves connected, through their beliefs and behaviour, to other people in the family system. This technique aimed to suggest and build relationships by the very process of questioning itself. The awareness of being in relationship opened the door for therapist and family members to see new connections, which created new contexts and meanings for the problem behaviour.

This final point, about finding new meaning in a new context, was a powerful feature of our work at the Tavistock because it also differentiated the Milan approach from others, which worked from a normative model of healthy functioning. We began to understand that people's behaviour in families was driven by meaning systems that were not universal but determined by each particular context. Instead of proposing that certain forms of family life were healthier than others, the Milan approach asserted that the normative view is a function of the position the therapist takes within a particular context that is part of the context of a larger system. For example, if my position is one of maintaining social control and child care standards, then I will match the family against normative standards agreed by myself and other social institutions; if, however, my position is one of a neutral therapist, I will try to loosen my grip on normative values and explore the 'local' meaning which families give to their own behaviour.

From 'I am different' to 'What are other people doing?'

As I look back over the development of both John's work and that of the Milan approach at the Tavistock, I am struck by the strategic importance of taking a particular point of view. For example, the development of family therapy as a respected mode of treatment within the Child and Family Department owes a great deal to John's early efforts to do something different in the department. Similarly, the development of the Milan approach would not have been possible if another group had not said, 'We are different.' We developed those aspects of the Milan approach that attracted us personally and conceptually, but we also clarified those features that distinguished us from other approaches within the family therapy team at that time.

Once we felt we had created an identity and space to work, e.g. through a family therapy qualification training course established in the mid-1980s by Ros Draper, Caroline Lindsey and myself, we were able to look further afield to see what other ideas or interests we might connect to. The same process was happening within the Milan team too. Those practitioners who were originally inspired or taught by Boscolo and Cecchin (Boscolo et al.,1980) used their ideas to interact with other people and other ideas in their own working contexts. I see this period in the mid-1980s as the beginning of the so-called post-Milan movement because it was a time in which the original ideas were re-examined from new perspectives or recast into new techniques for therapy and consulta-tion. For example, Karl Tomm in Calgary set out, in two highly influential papers, to describe how the Milan method works (Tomm, 1984a, 1984b). Interestingly, Boscolo and Cecchin, who collaborated with him, appreci-ated that Tomm could describe their work much better that they could! Tom Andersen, from the frozen tundra of north Norway, developed the Reflecting Team technique, which certainly expanded the concepts of neutrality and co-constructive therapy (Andersen, 1987). One ground-breaking paper critiqued the Milan approach from the feminist perspective, which opened a constructive debate about neutrality, therapeutic power and the difference between the political and therapeutic contexts (MacKinnon and Miller, 1987). In Britain, Ros Draper and I edited a book which included contributions from nearly 50 people who were all adapting the Milan systemic ideas to fit their various places of work (Campbell and Draper, 1985).

Current thinking and practice

It is inevitable that my version of post-Milan thinking will be influenced by the way I developed in the same time period and I want to guard against suggesting that everyone should be seeing things as I do. Since the introduction of the Milan approach in the early 1980s, I have seen many families, and discussed and supervised even more. I have become a more experienced and confident therapist, and I am more inclined to do whatever seems right for me at the time, rather than hold to one method in its correct form. Is this what happens to therapists as they get older? Probably. But on the other hand, as a trainer and teacher, I have to keep up with new thinking in order to give the trainees ideas which are 'of the current generation' as well as the ideas I have found helpful over the years. Therefore, it is from these positions that I offer my views about important ideas within the post-Milan movement and about the ideas which are, at the moment, important to me.

I have seen many trainees adopt various family therapy techniques, such as so-called circular questioning, without having the bigger picture of where these techniques were taking the therapy, and more seriously, without a full awareness of the ongoing relationship developing between themselves and their clients. The original four members of the Milan team were all very experienced psychoanalysts, before the idea of a circular question even entered their heads. Over the years that I have watched them working, I have been impressed by the quality of the client relationship, or the therapeutic alliance, as they conduct their interviews. I have often thought that the techniques of the Milan approach should be taught as advanced techniques, presented only after the therapist has developed the basic skills of listening empathetically and connecting with the client's feelings.

I think the field of family therapy is enriched by the revisiting of basic therapeutic concepts from the position of current ideas and techniques. For example, various people have taken a fresh look at psychoanalytic concepts, from the perspective of systemic thinking in the 1990s (Flaskas,

1993). I am interested to revisit the basic concept of the therapeutic relationship from the perspective of social constructionism and discourse psychology.

Talking about process

In order to create, with a client, a co-constructed therapeutic relationship, several things are important. The first is creating a context in which the evolving relationship can be talked about. For example, I would make it clear to clients that I want to be able to review with them the way our work together is going. I sometimes talk about 'ground rules', such as: I will need to hear from them if they think I am not being helpful in some way, perhaps I am asking questions which are too painful, or I may be skirting around issues which the family feels are more relevant. In order to do my part of the job I will probably want to support them in what they are trying to achieve but will also challenge them to look at some new ways of seeing things. Making therapy work requires communication back and forth about how we are working, as well as communication about the problems that have brought the clients to therapy.

Power

The second issue which I find helpful to address is the power differential between therapist and client. Co-construction should not suggest that two participants hold equal positions in the power hierarchy. The therapist is acknowledged, explicitly through professional training and job title, and implicitly through the choice of therapeutic interventions, as the person who has primary responsibility for the maintenance of the therapeutic work. The seeming paradox is that this responsibility, for an essentially interactional process, cannot be discharged without the full participation of clients. If one follows through the metaphor of the paradox, one could say: 'the therapist *is and is not* on an equal level with the clients'.

The implications for this are twofold: the therapist must not hold on to a mistaken belief about the presence of power, but rather acknowledge it and be aware of the myriad ways in which power shows itself in the therapy; and, secondly, to make this theme available as a topic for discussion, whenever appropriate, with the family.

Self-reflexivity

The third issue is related to self-reflexivity and the growing debate about the therapist's use of self (Boyd-Franklin, 1989; Flaskas, 1999). My particular aim is to raise awareness about the moments in therapy when I, as the therapist, am feeling pulled toward one point of view or I have a vague feeling that there is something else important that should be addressed but I cannot get to it. When doing live supervision, I often ask the therapist during a break: 'What do you think the family is doing to organize your thinking in one particular direction?' or, 'Do you have some ideas in the back of your mind which you feel you can't bring into the session?'

My basic premise as a supervisor is that once therapists develop a 'systemic frame of mind', it is the job of the supervisor to help the therapists become aware of their own obstacles which prevent them from listening and responding on the basis of their 'intuitions' and 'hunches'. I like the metaphor of the samurai warrior which Minuchin offered years ago: that is, therapists must train and train in the art of seeing systemic patterns, but when they are sitting down with the family, they must free themselves to respond to the family from their own natural, internal repertoire of responses.

Co-construction

The fourth point is about simultaneously holding firmly and loosely to one's ideas. Co-construction, at the cognitive level, is about creating a new idea or construct by resolving differences and, in order for this process to work, each party must feel free to take a position. Each must be able to say, 'I see it this way, and not that way.' I am opposed to the notion of absolute relativism whereby anything is as important as anything else. Rather, it is up to the therapist and client to create the best reality for themselves at that time, and then leave the door open, to allow themselves to be influenced to change their minds. This is accomplished by each side putting an idea forward i.e. 'holding firmly' and then becoming interested in the other person's response to the idea with the proviso that the original idea may very well be changed as a result of the ensuing conversation, i.e. 'holding loosely'. In this way, the process moves beyond the cognitive, 'in the-head', and on to the co-constructed space between people.

Representing the Other

I was struck by a paper I read several years ago entitled 'Theorizing Representing the Other' (Kitzinger and Wilkinson, 1996), in which the authors describe the way we put people in the position of being an 'other', any time we try to understand from our own perspective. An 'other' takes on the identity of being something we have actively placed in some position apart from ourselves, and which may therefore lose its opportunity to define itself. They cite the work of many writers who refer to the term 'othering' to identify this process. This process has powerful implications for both therapy and research, where there is such a high premium placed on understanding, conceptualizing and describing. If it is not possible to do therapy without 'othering' our clients, and silencing their voices, perhaps we can become more aware of our part in this process.

If we take the othering process seriously, it seem to me therapists will need to reconsider the assumptions underlying the narrative approach to therapy and, perhaps, change the way therapy is conducted. One of Michael White's invaluable contributions to the family therapy field has been the introduction, supported by the writings of Foucault, of the notion of a dominant story that governs our lives and the alternative story that remains untold (White, 1995). In *Re-Authoring Lives: Interviews and Essays*, he states:

> In the work that I have been discussing here, there is at times a renaming of the dominant plot, but always a naming of a counterplot or alternative plot. This process of renaming and naming is really important. The naming of an alternative plot greatly facilitates the ascription of meaning to a whole range of experiences that have previously been neglected.

However, the questions remain: who is the author of the new narrative and what is the process by which the final narrative is created? Does a client create the new narrative and reach a new sense of self, which ultimately defines a 'self' in relation to an 'other'? Are these the best conceptual tools for family therapists? Developing a new sense of self may be crucial for individuals and for a therapy that is based on helping an individual in the context of a family, but family therapists need tools that emphasize difference and interaction between family members rather than the more boundaried concept of self. (I may be doing narrative therapists an injustice here: they must be able to take clients on a journey that looks at the interaction of many different stories of self to reach the final destination. I have done this work myself with some clients to good effect.)

The dialogical self

Several authors have introduced me to the concept of the dialogical self. Bakhtin, the Russian literary critic and philosopher (Bakhtin, 1981) and Edward Sampson (Sampson, 1993) a contemporary American psychologist, are part of a larger movement that challenges traditional narrative theory and shifts the emphasis to exploring the various patterns that develop between the self and other. These ideas can potentially help therapists to develop new tools for therapy which are based on interactional systemic thinking.

Bakhtin creates a dichotomy between identity, which is coherent, and difference, which is disorder, and he states that it is difference rather than identity that is necessary for understanding. He bases his philosophy on the contrary forces which are inherent in language; every word or utterance represents a point where two forces are brought together. There is a centripetal force which brings this word together with other similar words and tends toward agreement and unity. A sentence such as 'it is raining' contains a force which brings together other similar words and experiences to create meaning; but the same sentence also contains a centrifugal force which seeks difference, disagreement and multiple views, inviting thoughts about good weather and sunshine.

He proposes that a dialogical self is not based, like a narrative self, on coherence and unity but that it knows itself through the contrary tensions within language which mirror the contraries within our minds. The dialogical self knows itself through the response of 'other' because the other creates the contrary forces. This is a compelling justification for keeping the 'other', whether it be real or imaginary, past, present or future, alive in the therapeutic conversations we create with clients. The narrative approach has interested me for a number of years because of the rewarding pleasure of releasing a buried part of the client's self. It is a powerful technique with individual clients but I have struggled to find ways to bring these ideas into the family therapy arena. One of the ways in which family members can experience a dialogical self is through externalising the problem (White, 1989). In the case I am going to present, a young boy, in the midst of family therapy, is able to explore the way his 'symptom' is both unifying for the family but also creating great tensions which threaten to break things further apart.

A case illustration

My own style as a family therapist is eclectic and like many post-Milan therapists I use different techniques at different stages of therapy. I have chosen to present this particular case because attachment is at the heart of the work and various ideas and techniques employed that helped family members to leave their attachments behind. In this case, I have organized the presentation into four stages, each of which represents a different therapeutic position or technique within the broadening spectrum of post-Milan family therapy.

Paul, aged 9, was referred because he developed acute anxiety states about his mother's safety when they were separated. This led to continuous phone calls to check that she was alright and to agreements about the precise time mother would return home. Paul would begin to watch for her a few minutes before the expected time of arrival and, if she were merely a minute late, would collapse in a state of anxiety and hyperventilation. Paul was the elder of two children, with a sister aged 7, in a family that had been through a painful divorce several years earlier. The children lived with their mother but saw their father frequently, and both parents had new partners.

Stage 1: Letting the family tell their story

The whole family was invited to the first session. I wanted simply to let them talk about what they were feeling. There was a great deal of tension between mother and father who sat at opposite sides of the room. As we talked about the divorce, the family became very tearful and the children moved to sit on their parents' laps. It seemed as though the divorce had only happened yesterday. It struck me that Paul was very resentful about the new partners. He didn't like it when he was with a parent and the other partner tried to be friendly, as though the partner wanted this new unit 'to be like a family'.

I purposely tried not to think too much but rather to empathize with what the different family members were going through and to share enough of this to reassure them that I would try to respect and hold in mind their experiences while we were working together.

This piece of work with the family is not described in conceptual terms. It is more 'from the heart' if you will. Many Milan therapists, myself included, have been enamoured in the past with systemic formulations and interviewing techniques. This was necessary at the time to develop a new model but these therapists are now more explicit about integrating their empathy and personal responses into their therapeutic work.

Stage 2: Exploring systemic hypotheses

I organized my thoughts around two hypotheses: Paul had been a central lynchpin between his parents, in this closely knit, affectionate family, and he was losing some of the closeness to each parent, as well as the powerful role of being a 'switchboard' in the family. But adding the systemic perspective, i.e. looking at how others contribute to the problem behaviour, I surmised that the parents felt personally uncertain about moving to the next stage of their lives, so it may have been difficult to give the children clear messages about the new partners. I also sensed that they felt terrible about inflicting so much pain on their children through the divorce, and perhaps there was an embargo on angry and blaming feelings that usually accompany divorce. One could see how the problem behaviour might be experienced by the family as holding things back from further development, and diverting feelings of anger or despair into more acceptable feelings of concern and closeness.

We explored these themes. I explained to the family that I thought it would be helpful to have some understanding of what was going on for all of them, in order to give some possible meaning to why the family was in this predicament. I had some ideas I wanted to discuss with them, but this was not all we would do to tackle the problem. I also wanted to work directly with them to help Paul get this behaviour under control so he could also get on with his life.

Stage 3: Externalizing the problem

After several sessions, the father was unable to attend a series of meetings because of work commitments, so I used this opportunity to shift my focus and work with Paul and his mother. My intention was to describe a pattern and purpose in Paul's behaviour and to give it a name that he could identify, and to which we could both refer during our future conversations. He chose to call it his 'worry'. The next step was to describe the 'worry' as an external force outside himself – a powerful force with a life of its own which, for its own reasons, lands on him from time to time causing him to worry about his parents' safety. Paul liked this discussion and got involved drawing a picture of 'worry' as a red cloud. But before I could elicit his resistance to worry, I needed to draw out examples from his own life of fighting back against forces intended to defeat him. In the first session Paul had said he was very keen on football and an avid Tottenham Hotspur supporter, so I explored this area to find examples of how he would fight back on the football pitch if someone took the ball away from him.

Once this was clearly established, we worked together to identify a series of strategies he could use to fight against the worry and keep it at bay for a brief period each day. We went through each day of the week to identify when and how the worry landed on him. For example, on Mondays Paul went to a neighbour's after school until his mother returned from work. His usual pattern was to walk into the neighbour's house and go straight to the telephone to call his mother. We externalized this process by saying 'worry' was waiting for him at the neighbour's front door and landed on his shoulder the moment he walked in, which caused him to rush to the telephone. Paul agreed that he could try to keep worry at bay by postponing the phone call to his mother for one minute by taking off his coat and speaking briefly to the neighbour when he arrived, but after 60 seconds he was to go straight to the telephone to contact his mother as usual.

In the context of systemic family work, it was possible, in this case, to enlist the support of Paul's parents, and even the neighbour, to help him keep worry at bay by both respecting his attempts to resist it, and also his need to let it control him and guide his actions. The adults knew about

Paul's weekly strategy and were aware that they should support his efforts but not expect too much too soon, nor take any of the initiative away from Paul – he was engaged in his own personal struggle with worry and would slowly overcome it in his way and in his time.

Together, Paul, his mother and I designed a weekly plan in which Paul would keep worry at bay for one minute each day. The circumstances were different each day – some days, for example, he would be with his father, others alone at home with his sister – so we had to be creative about the best strategies for each situation and the best way to involve others to support his plan. Doing this detailed work over several sessions clarified Paul's strategy but, also, the slow methodical discussion of worry in all its week-long manifestations seemed to have the effect of exposing its mystery and loosening its grip on Paul. As our sessions continued, Paul lost some interest in these strategies, as though he was getting bored with the process and wanted to think about other things. This also coincided with his success with the strategies and the gradual expansion from one minute to two then three minutes during which he could keep worry at bay.

After four sessions dedicated to this work both Paul and his mother felt there had been considerable improvement. The problem was not so controlling of their lives and they felt they could carry on with the weekly plans on their own. Toward the end of this period, Paul decided he would be able to go on a week-long school trip to Wales. We discussed how he would deal with 'worry', who might become more powerful when Paul was so far from home, and the family discussed their own strategies which included asking his grandfather to buy him a pager for the trip!

Stage 4: Individual work in the family context

The final stage of my work was initiated by Paul himself. At the beginning of the fifth session, Paul's mother said he wanted to have a meeting with me on his own. He had always been reticent and cautious during the family meetings and I was very curious why he wished to talk with me now. I agreed to end the family meeting early so he could have half the session with me.

When we were alone he launched straight into a story. One evening, several years earlier, he answered the telephone to hear a female voice crying and saying, 'I'm having an affair.' This left Paul very confused about whether this was a prank or a true story and, if it was true, who was this woman, and what would it mean to him and his own explanation for the reason his parents split up?

Two issues interested me particularly as Paul and I unravelled his story. One was the deep sense of hurt and outrage that his father might have been having an affair. Paul sounded to me like a jilted lover. I wondered if he had some idea that his close relationship with his mother was like an affair that excluded his father. (Some therapists would describe this as a hypothesis about oedipal rivalry.) When children are entwined with adult relationships that they do not understand, it is very difficult to come to terms with a divorce, and probably doubly difficult if there are underground secret relationships. I discussed this theme by asking for his own explanation as to why his parents split up, adding that children often have two explanations: one is 'sensible', and a second one, which is more weird and confusing, in which they think they are partly responsible for the break-up. He agreed that he was very confused and we continued to talk about how he had always fitted in between his parents.

The second issue became clearer to me when I asked myself why Paul wanted to have this private session. In terms of the previous hypothesis, one could speculate that he wanted to retain a secret relationship with his mother, but I was struck by his reply when I asked him if he saw his mother as a fragile person. He immediately said, 'Yes', with a look of recognition that I had not seen on his face before. This led me to explore the hypothesis that Paul was deeply worried about whether his mother would survive the break-up. Many of the things that were on his mind might hurt her further; this struck a chord with Paul and we discussed it at length. I tried to empathize with his dilemma that on the one hand he might like his mother to have a new partner for support in her life but, on the other hand, that would mean a new man intruding into his relationship with his mother.

After a second session divided between the family and a time for Paul, his mother suggested things had improved and they didn't feel they needed further meetings. Paul wanted to know if he could have a final session with his father. During this meeting, I was struck by the way Paul explained how badly he felt about staying in his father's house and about his partner, and by the way his father patiently and reasonably listened to the catalogue of complaints. Something didn't seem right but I couldn't put my finger on it. It finally occurred to me that this process seemed to mask more dangerous, angry feelings about the break-up and we spent most of the session talking about how difficult it was to have these feelings of anger and sadness, and perhaps Paul wanted to try to be strong by building up power and control in his life and the lives of his parents.

We said goodbye after this session. I told them to contact me again if they thought further meetings would be helpful, but I have not heard from them in the six months since that time.

Conclusion

I hope the reader can see from this chapter that John's passion for family therapy and his ability to stand up for a different approach, helped create the space within the Tavistock for the development of the first training course in the UK, and subsequently for the development of new therapists with their own brands of therapy. The field has moved beyond the stage in which clearly defined schools of therapy jostled for prominence, yet his contribution to family therapy theory and practice will endure because he found a way to transform his lifelong interest in family stories into powerful therapeutic techniques. I frequently hear therapists describing the ways they explore replicative and corrective scripts with their client families. I remember John once describing his role as a therapist as a person to whom his clients will make a strong attachment at the beginning of therapy and gradually become less attached to him and more attached to family relationships or the outside world. Working alongside John for 25 years was an education in itself and I count myself one among the many clinicians in the field who have absorbed, by osmosis, his ideas about attachment and family scripts.

This case illustration was also used in an article entitled: Family Therapy and Beyond: Where is the Milan Systemic Approach Today? Child Psychology and Psychiatry Review. (Campbell, 1999)

David Campbell is a Consultant Clinical Psychologist in the Child and Family Department at the Tavistock Clinic in London, where he is teaches and supervises for the Masters course in Family Therapy and the Doctorate in Systemic Psychotherapy. His research interests lie in the field of childhood depression and the users' experience of family therapy. Apart from his clinic work he is also a freelance organizational consultant, specializing in team building and strategic planning for teams and small organizations in the public sector. David is the co-editor of a series of books entitled the Systemic Thinking and Practice Series (Karnac Books). His latest contribution to this series is Socially Constructed Organisation *(Karnac Books, 2000). He is married to a language teacher and has two children in the stages of leaving home. His hobbies include looking for free time, and gardening and cycling when he finds it.*

Chapter 4
Families and child psychotherapy: a Kleinian perspective

JEANNE MAGAGNA

Introduction

In the 1890s my Italian grandmother, aged 18, emigrated to a coal-mining village in the USA. She was fiercely religious, considering it 'a sin' to read the Bible of another faith. As soon as I could walk, I was her 'little shadow' accompanying her everywhere she went. I adored her. However, when I was five years old, my parents moved from the extended family residence to a house of their own. The new house, with my young and beautiful mother, was filled with American comforts, including the television when it reached our small town. Outdoor life provided a freedom for the children who played in the nearby sagebrush dessert, unsupervised, from the age of six.

By the time I was an adolescent, I felt terribly grown-up and entitled to wear the make-up, high heels, flouncy skirts typical of the 1950s woman like my mother. From the age of 14, the adolescents, myself included, also drove their hot-rods and second-hand cars to school and regularly spent Friday and Saturday night dancing in the high-school gymnasium. My grandmother, Nona, as I called her, was very critical of my new-found adolescence. She did this partially because she could not appreciate the difference between my social life, which included boys, and her Italian adolescence, characterized by prayer, church attendance and hard work. If I loved her, I should follow her ideals for a young girl.

In the late 1960s, some eight years after leaving my little town in Wyoming, I found myself embarking on the child psychotherapy training at the Tavistock Clinic. As I was doing my child psychotherapy training, family therapy conferences with Salvador Minuchin and Peggy Papp were absorbing the interest of some of the talented child psychiatrists at the Tavistock Clinic, including John Byng-Hall. The child psychotherapy programme seemed to look rather scathingly at the new family therapy approaches which included using the one-way screen, live supervision with a 'bug in one ear', and meeting with the whole family regularly, rather than spending regular time alone with the identified patient. Salvador Minuchin's approach, which involved humour, moving around in the room, challenging and giving directives, seemed spontaneous and extroverted compared to my overly restrained version of 'proper psychoanalytic technique' for a child psychotherapist.

As I kept my hand on the pulse of the family therapy movement and maintained my presence in the child psychotherapy seminars, I felt gripped by sensations similar to those I felt when experiencing the ideological conflicts represented by my modern American mother and my beloved 'old country' Nona. Who was right? Which idea of moving forward as a therapist was 'better'? There was no doubt an unacknowledged competition between the growing 'family therapist group' and the more traditional 'child psychotherapy group' at the Tavistock Clinic. When I matured from my position as a student, what kind of a 'grown-up therapist' would I become?

Growing up and learning from experience is a difficult and painful process, always filled with some failure. A child with mother and grandmother in conflict has a perfect opportunity for projecting unwanted aspects of herself into them. Likewise, as a student, I could project my inadequacies and use my thwarted aggressive critical voice as I encountered the realms of the family therapists and the child psychotherapists. In the 1970s there seemed to be no space for being a child psychotherapist *and* a family therapist.

Sitting in the seminars of either group made me feel very uncomfortable in relation to the other group. Certainly it didn't seem 'proper' to have a child both in ongoing family therapy as well as in intensive child psychotherapy. It was considered 'too confusing' for the child to have more than one therapist with different work being done and different transferences to each therapist. Child psychotherapy would 'spoil' the systemic work of the family therapist, and family therapy was considered to 'disrupt' the work of the individual child psychotherapist. These comments were voiced regularly in family and child psychotherapy camps. 'Growing up' involved the anxiety of being unfaithful to my grandmother or my mother. Similarly, devising my ideal way of working with children and their families brought the same risk.

Accepting what feels therapeutically useful

Like my father, who was the link because he respected the views of both my paternal grandmother and my American mother, John Byng-Hall became 'my bridge' between child psychotherapy and family therapy. For six years we invited him to supervise our work regularly with families in the Royal Free Hospital Child Psychiatry Department, located a few minutes away from the Tavistock Clinic. I later formally completed the Sheldon Fellow Family Therapy Programme with his supervision.

John was a wonderful 'bridge' because he, like my father, had the capacity to experience conflict, absorb the tension, think about what was essential and then speak sparingly about 'the central issues'. He could stand alone, with his own Byng-Hall approach to families. He has had the courage to risk being called 'the unfashionable John-Byng Hall' (Larner, 1999). His approach seemed to reflect no popular family therapy 'technique of the day', but rather his own integration of therapeutically useful approaches derived from John Bowlby's work, family therapy and child psychoanalytic psychotherapy, all of which existed at the Tavistock Clinic where he worked. Withstanding the pressure to 'fit into' a particular model, John remained a bridge that allowed the current of creativity to flow through him and inform his humour, his warmth and his artistic vision. Allowing us to share his innovative work with families, his own landscape paintings and anecdotes from his own family were part of his generous style.

Working with 'the bug in the ear', John's voice made me feel a much better therapist than I actually was. I felt conflicted about this at times intrusive style of supervision; however, being more immediately able to function well with a family was useful for building my self-confidence as a therapist.

Work with a family illustrating integration of child psychotherapy and John Byng-Hall's approach to families

I shall illustrate my appreciation of John's approach by presenting the family work which he supervised. My aim will be to demonstrate how John enabled me to make an internal bridge between my psychoanalytic training and his approach to work with families. In particular I will show how John facilitated the creation of a space for valuing young children's spontaneous verbal and nonverbal communications in family therapy sessions.

Hypothesis about the symptom

Several families were referred with a latency-aged child presenting night-terrors and nightmares. This gave me a perfect opportunity to look at both the night-time internalized family relationships and the day-time external family relationships. Looking at both the nightmare and dream life of family members and their external relationships, I was able to formulate the hypothesis that night terrors and nightmares in latency-aged children are found in families where a child is paralysed in an incestuous triangulation in the parental relationship and denial of hostility is a shared family defence.

The children and the family's dream-life provide mental containers for unsettling feelings and unwanted parts of the self (Handler, 1972). Infant observation on a regular basis, which forms part of the child psychotherapy training, enabled me to see how the baby holds parts of the mother's anxiety that she looks after in her baby. Within the context of the family therapy session, watching the children play, suggesting that children draw and allowing family members to share some dreams, allowed access to the unexpressed conflicts and anxieties present in the family.

Had I seen the six-year-old boy with night-terrors in individual therapy, I would have missed the fact that as part of the larger family system mother and son were engaged in mutually seductive activities which fostered disturbance in both the boy and his mother. Sleeping with mother, taking the place of father in bed with mother, and cuddling with her created a 'blurring of generational boundaries' and chronic sexual overstimulation of the young boy. However, there had not been sufficient interest in this quasi-incestuous relationship between mother and son because overtly the mother was simply calming her frightened child. A child psychotherapist viewing the difficulty might say that some of the mother's chronic anxiety had been displaced unto her child and she tried to comfort it in him. But John augmented this understanding by suggesting that the partnership between the parents was such that mother was not coupled with her husband in such a way that he could receive his wife's anxieties and support her. I realized that structural family therapy on its own would do nothing to change this incestuous pairing. Dr Leo Rangell (1950), a noted therapist, discovered that despite repeated requests to parents to work together to keep the child out of the bedroom, the parents frequently slept with the child and hid the fact from the therapist.

The child as a marital distance regulator or 'the terrifying triangle'

When a child has passed into latency he should, under normal circumstances, have developed a sufficient internal container or, in other words, sufficient ego-strength, to be able to sleep and dream through the night. Therefore, I assume that the terror-producing situations probably have a basis in the psychic reality of the family. John's (Byng-Hall, 1980) classic paper, 'The Symptom Bearer as a Marital Distance Regulator', helped me to avoid focusing initially on the marital relationship. He suggested that the boy with night-terrors might be functioning as a shared protective mechanism by the parents and warned that couples quickly take flight if the therapist takes away their defence of the symptomatic child too quickly.

But he didn't stop me from wondering silently about how the paralysis of the child in the night terrors, which does not allow him to flee successfully from the objects of terror, relates to an actual paralysis of a child caught inside the mother and father's marital relationship. I thought that perhaps one or both of the parents had trapped him in his particular role as a defence against marital anxieties. The boy's own oedipal longings and resultant night-time anxieties augmented the pressure for him to remain 'next to mother in bed' and 'between the marital couple'.

Providing a secure, dependable setting for therapeutic work to take place

A central feature of the child psychotherapy training is an acknowledgement that the family members bring not only the mature aspects of their personalities into play in the session, but also the more infantile aspects, the 'baby-self', into a potentially dependent relationship with the therapist. Observing a four-month-old infant with its mother provides a poignant picture of how the mothering figure's presence can bring joy while her absence can create disappointment and distress until the infant has internalized a secure inner base, a good 'containing mother' (Magagna, 1987).

Example

> Mother comes into the room and sits behind baby. Baby turns her head to the right and cranes her neck and head backwards in a rather awkward position in order to see mother. Mother, while talking on the phone, gives baby a big smile and baby grins back, excitedly flaps her arms up and down a couple of times while kicking her legs out straight out and up and down on the mattress. Baby then reaches to take hold of one of mother's fingers from the hand extended near baby's head. She strains her head to keep taking a look at mother's face. A few minutes later, mother puts a pacifier into baby's mouth and walks out of the room. Baby follows her with her eyes and continually looks in the direction of mother whose voice can still be heard talking on the mobile phone. Then baby spits the pacifier which literally flies up into the air before falling down. Baby then spreads her arms out, like a bird with wings outspread and then thumps the arms down against her sides. Her legs go straight out in front of her, her toes curl in and out and she bumps her feet against one another. Mother walks by and out through another door, she goes out of baby's hearing. Baby then stretches her arms above her head and her whole body goes completely limp. Shortly, she furrows her brow and lets out a cry. When mother returns, baby waves her arms and kicks her legs excitedly as she smiles at mother and takes some deep breaths.

Doing a baby observation, weekly for two years, and seeing how intense and enduring the infant's dependence is on the relationship with the mother had an immense impact on me. I became fully convinced of how important it was to acknowledge the infantile dependence which accompanies more mature aspects of the family's relationship with the therapist. If infant observation were central to the family therapy trainings, it would certainly modify premature focusing on parents' parenting skills and adult coping selves while ignoring the effects of the presence and absence of the therapist.

I attempt to provide a setting with as much predictability and reliability in it as possible. Part of my 'predictable setting' includes fortnightly sessions at a regular time for one hour. Acknowledging the gaps created by my lack of understanding of certain aspect of the family, the separations between the sessions and preparing for holidays all represent some of my attempts to establish a 'secure setting' for the family. The children retain exclusive use of the family box of simple play materials including paper, crayons, plasticine, family dolls, a few families of animals and some cars. All the children's drawings are saved in a folder and brought to each session as a kind of 'history book' which can be used in subsequent family sessions. The play area is designated as being in the centre on a small table. I avoid tempting the children out of the safe, visible, central play arena by excluding the use of toys in other parts of the room. The certainty of having the same therapy room and the predictability of other aspects of their relationship with me enables the family to develop enough dependence to feel secure enough to explore their innermost difficulties. I say this, acknowledging that it is the trustworthiness of the therapist and not only the helpful interventions of the therapist that are important.

Gathering of the family's 'total transference' to the institution and the therapist

John's work on John Bowlby's attachment theory promoted his appreciation of children's distressed response to lack of a secure attachment to parenting figures. Although he did not encourage me to make interpretations around the family's responses to separation and mismatches in communication, he encouraged and allowed me to find my own bridge between child psychotherapy and family therapy. I felt it was important to focus not primarily on the historical past or family processes outside the session. I was interested in gathering the whole of the family's transference to the setting, the institutional procedures and my interpretations. This gathering of the transference to me, the therapist, initially tended to lessen the emotional burden of the parents. They were already stressed by the presenting symptom. Through accepting the family's dependence on me I was sharing some of the intensity of feeling and worrying anxieties present in the family.

Focus on anxieties in the immediate present

My task, which is central to Kleinian child psychotherapy, is to focus on the family members' emotions that are most immediate and pressing in the experience of the therapy session. Underlying this is the idea that internal change in the family could be helpfully facilitated by encouraging both the parents and their children to use both their mature understanding and supportive capacities to meet anxiety, face psychic conflict and bear psychic pain at the moment they are being experienced in the session. The family's spontaneous remarks alongside their non-verbal communication, the children's drawing, behaviour and play are all used to find ways of helping the family members resolve their conflicts.

Supporting the healthy more mature aspects of the family members

John helped me to resolve some of the confusion resulting from seeing group therapy and psychoanalytic family therapy in practice, where there was more of a focus on the infantile anxieties and conflicts of each of the family members. Although I focused on the relationships existing between the family members and between the family and me, he helped me to realize that the parents needed to be brought back into the parenting position with the child in his 'child' position before certain therapeutic endeavours would be safe to pursue. In other words, the children needed to see some difference in my way of relating to their parents as having more adult responsibility for meeting the children's emotional pressures. It was important that not every family member was treated as being at the same developmental level in my eyes.

Through John I also began to realize how I could support and facilitate the parenting capacity of the parents valuing and emphasizing their strengths. Previously my personal and strange version of psychoanalysis seemed to focus more on conflicts and repressed feelings of the patients. Not only did John change my work with families, but his acknowledgement of the strengths in the family members and his positively connoting different aspects of family behaviour (Byng-Hall, 1986) radically altered my individual psychoanalytic work. In particular, I realize now that it is essential to mobilize the ego strengths of traumatised and borderline patients and empathize with the original protective function of certain symptoms.

Working with the families of children experiencing night terrors and nightmares

My integration of family therapy and psychoanalytic child psychotherapy techniques led me to adopt the following approach in working with these families where the children couldn't sleep because of disturbing night-life experiences:

1. Using structural methods to help parents work together in combining their roles of nurturing and providing parental authority, while at the same time acknowledging their own infantile needs.
2. Helping the family members understand their patterns of interaction which were observable at that moment in the session.
3. Assisting the family to gain the capacity to experience rather than evade the intrapsychic emotional conflicts.
4. Fostering an appreciation for the children's drawing, behaviour and play as the medium through which they primarily expressed and worked through anxieties relating to the family dynamics occurring in the immediate present of the session.

'Joining' with all family members while exploring the purpose of the clinic visit

Trevarthen (1979) made it impressively clear that when child psychotherapists greeted patients for the first time, their traditional presentation of themselves as being 'neutral', that is not smiling in a friendly way, was actually experienced as unfriendly and a deprivation of the ordinary human way of greeting another person. John's approach to families was my first experience of a psychotherapeutic mode of greeting the family that felt 'people friendly'. But more importantly, he also 'joined' with me, his supervisee, in such a way that I was able to feel supported as I established with the family an emotional link which fostered love, acknowledged hostility and provided security sufficient to bear the unbearable truths. The family feel the quality of the supervisee's relationship with the supervisor, just as children feel the parents' relationship with one another.

Before giving the children in the family access to play materials, I explore with parents and the children what the children know about why they are coming to the clinic. Respecting the children's experience of being at the clinic is extremely important to me. Too often I have felt that 'the adults' keep the children as 'inferior beings' who are left to feel humiliated as the parents complain about the children's problematic behaviour.

Example of joining family with night terrors

The Cuddle family, consisting of four children, came to the clinic. Daniel (10), Shirley (8), Jack (6) and Kismet (3) all said they had come to discuss the problem of six-year-old Jack who experienced night-terrors. All the children and the parents took part in the discussion, with the children often trying to interrupt their parents in order to contribute. The children indicated that Jack was frightened of a daddy long legs, the BFG (big friendly giant) on television and the dark. I asked who else was worried about them. Several of the children said that they too were frightened of these things. Various children drew pictures of family members which are below:

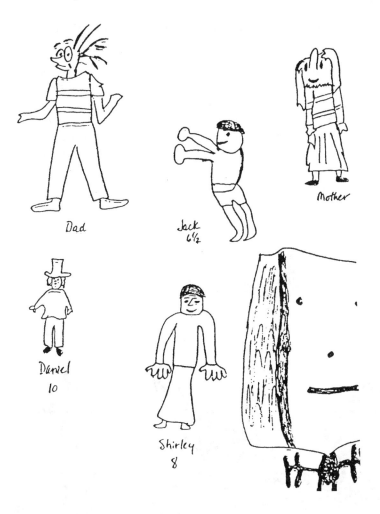

Figure 4.1 Family members: drawings by various children.

The parents responded to Jack's fear of being alone at night by allowing him to sleep with them. Much of the time during the session Jack was lying sideways in his mother's lap, like a young baby, sucking his finger. He said he would like to be an elf. At other times he was hugging mother, hitting his head against her breasts. Later he hit his dad, then hugged him, and then shouted, 'I don't like you' to him. In a subsequent session Jack drew a boy falling into the water while saying, 'This is terrible.' The boy was then drawn immersed in the water, shouting for help while drowning among the sharks. Someone was rowing out to save the boy saying, 'I'm coming.' I described how there was this nameless fear around in the night – like drowning in the night – and the family hoped that I could help them with this.

Sharing my hypothesis about the function of the night terror symptom

If I had been treating Jack in individual therapy I might have been looking at his oedipal wishes and resultant anxieties in his relationship with 'the mother', as represented by the therapist in the transference. However, in working with this family, John had fostered my appreciation of the usefulness of a symptom. This was quite a different viewpoint for me, but it transformed my approach in assessing a child's suitability for individual child psychotherapy. Now I always precede any work with an individual child by working briefly with the family and insisting that parental work or family work always accompanies individual therapy with a family member.

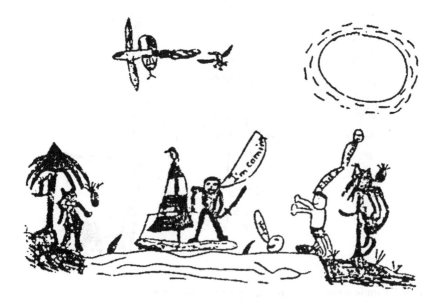

Figure 4.2 Boy drowning: drawing by Jack.

Example of describing the usefulness of the symptom

> At the end of the first session with the Cuddle family I asked the parents to have the children return to their chairs to hear me deliver my hypothesis about the function of the symptom night terrors. I said that Jack, by being so frightened with night terrors, was enabling the parents to come together at the clinic to help him. Coming to the clinic also enabled help to be given to the other children who are also triangulated into helping and protecting their parents. Cuddling with mother at night enables her to give and receive physical affection.

Helping parents work together

The beauty of the structural model of work with parents is that it facilitates them to use their own therapeutic parenting capacities, rather than presenting an idea that they, like their child, have difficulties requiring therapy. However, when the couple are not able to support each other and meet each other's emotional needs, they tend to feel the therapist's request to do even more for the family as a virtually impossible drain on their emotional resources. It is for this reason that I focus first on what the parents feel they each require to go forward with the difficult task of helping their children with the difficulties they are experiencing.

Example

> Mother's need for a supportive partner came out when she said she did not want to be a big powerful woman who did what her husband should do and had to tell him to do it. We looked at her difficulties in asking for help and she tried out different ways of calling on father to help her before she was at her wits' end. Father said he would feel better if he did not end up always being the disciplinarian. Both expressed hostility both to each other and to me for not meeting their needs. By gathering some of their hostility into the transference to me, I felt I mitigated some of the sharpness of their hostility to each other for not meeting each other's needs.

Following a strictly psychoanalytic technique would have never involved me in giving suggestions for action, such as making a sleep chart for Jack and asking the parents actively to make decisions about where Jack was to sleep at night, rather than letting him dominate their authority with his night fears. John Byng-Hall was making suggestions for me to ask the parents to do things. Initially, I felt resistant to change 'my style'. Making a change involved anxiety about losing some of my clearly established identity as a 'psychoanalytic psychotherapist'. I had been clinging onto this identity for a sense of personal security.

I realized to my amazement that if the family is in a positive transference to the therapist, following a suggestion for supporting one another or being firm with the children creates an opportunity for practice in being someone different from who one usually is. Sometimes experiencing the effectiveness of 'being' and 'acting' in a different way from usual can feel a relief to a parent who feels at his or her wits' end. I also realized that if they were in a negative transference, the couple was resistant to any structural work involving the nurturing the children and being firm with the children. I needed to work through negativity towards me for not under-standing the couple's primary concerns before I could proceed.

Focusing on 'secret' worries of the family

I told the family that my experience was that when things were out in the open, children are much more able to deal with the family secrets. A dialogue began between the children and myself about the anxiety-laden, non-verbal images which the children brought to the session.

Example

On one occasion, when the parents were particularly unforthcoming, Jack, 6, and Shirley, 8 , started giggling together and then ran to hide behind separate chairs. Jack called out to Shirley not to look and Shirley repeated 'Don't look.' In their excited pairing they revealed their understanding that they were not to know about some frightening family secret.

Later in the session Daniel began drawing a picture of a man with blackened eyes. When he finished the picture, I began discussing it with him, hoping to use it in relating to the shared anxieties of the family. He said that the man had black airport glasses on. He was telling the plane to go. The pilot had to taken off, but somebody said 'Shut up'. There were signs on his drawing saying 'Go-go-go' and signs saying 'Shut-up'. I talked to the whole family about the dilemma raised in Daniel's drawing: should we talk about what was happening or did we have to remain 'shut up'?

After a pause, I commented that everyone has worries and asked what might the other family worries be besides Jack's night terrors. Three-year-old Kismet replied immediately, 'Mummy and Daddy are upset!' When I asked if that was all that worried her she said 'Yes'. I wondered aloud about how perhaps all the children shared her worry. I thought perhaps they might want to talk about how they each responded to their mummy and daddy being upset. Daniel, 10, said his father was working in a factory and did not have a proper 'wench'. There was a basket of bricks hanging and Daniel was worried that the rope would crash on his father's head and then his dad would not come home safely.

Later Daniel asked his parents, 'Why don't you divorce?' When I asked who might be worried about that happening, Daniel quickly answered that he was not worried, because he had asked his mummy if she was going to get divorced and she promised him she would not. I commented that perhaps someone was worried about mummy and daddy separating and losing daddy and Daniel retorted, 'Who wouldn't?'

The night terrors seemed to reflect the family's uncertainty about the marriage breaking up, the insecurity accompanying this uncertainty. John

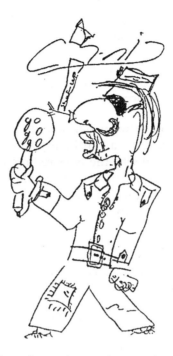

Figure 4.3 Man with blackened eyes: drawing by Daniel.

(Byng-Hall, 1995a) has written extensively on creating a secure family base and helped me to understand how the children probably felt the secret about the marriage conflict and potential break-up was more frightening because they felt the parents were not secure enough to talk about it.

> I described how the parents were faced with the dilemma of what to do with 'the other things' they did not want to talk about. They felt that not talking to the children about these things might protect them, but I had another idea. I thought children felt secrets are more horrific. The children might feel that it was impossible to speak about something if it was really terrible. Father responded that their children knew a lot from observing, but they needed someone to help them in making sense of what they were picking up. Mother answered quickly that it was confusion.

Using dramatization and drawings for the safe expression of hostility and interpretation as a reparative act

Denying a problem and keeping it a secret because it is too painful to face is a pattern typical of families where a member has night terrors. This family's secret was that father had bought a flat in a nearby city and had a new partner. The parents did separate. The children were then more anxious about acknowledging their hostile feelings for fear that they had caused the break-up through their oedipal longings and the emotional burden they placed on the couple.

> In one session the children showed me what happened at home. Daniel and Jack began sitting on top of one another fighting and Shirley, 8, pretended to be in her bedroom stamping her feet because she was angry.

I used this dramatization of what happened at home to highlight the hostility which the children had difficulty openly acknowledging to mother. I explored how and why the boys redirected their anger towards mother to each other in their fighting. I used Shirley's feet stomping as a reason for providing special time in the session for Shirley and mother to look at their fraught relationship.

> Then Daniel drew a picture:
> Daniel drew this picture of murderers with blackened sunglasses to stop them from seeing the victim whom they are about to murder. I described how Daniel and the other children were trying to find a safe place for their anger. I added that Daniel was expressing the whole family's anxiety: if they acknowledged their hostility towards each other and the parents, they feared the anger was so strong it would only destroy someone or send them away, like dad was 'sent away' in their minds. I told them that much of the time they felt they had to hide their anger among themselves.

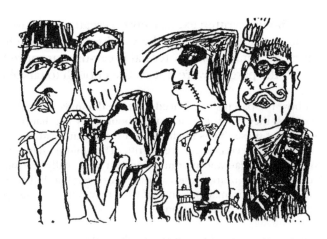

Figure 4.4 Five murderers: drawing by Daniel.

> Daniel continued to express the precarious family situation through the family life boat which was broken through the middle.
> I talked about the boat cracking through the torpedo of hostility and shock at the parents' marital break-up during the holiday, accompanied by my absence. I described how therapy and the family with the parents together was a lifeboat

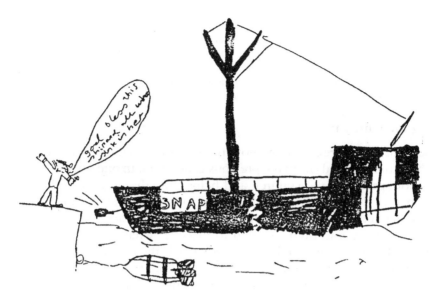

Figure 4.5 Boat cracking in the middle: drawing by Daniel.

supporting the family, but now they felt this secure 'lifeboat' had been cracked. I noted all the sexual posturing, including laying on top of each other and French kissing between Jack and Kismet at difficult moments during the session. I talked about their having to cling intensely together because they were so frightened to be separate and so anxious about the shocking news of mother and dad living apart.

Making a 'family friends chart'

The children experienced themselves as being 'too much' for mother and worried about her survival and/or her sending them away to boarding school. Because of this, they tended to cling to her and bury their grievances which they needed to express to feel understood and supported by mother and me. John prompted me to get down on the floor with the children and have them make a 'family friends' chart'. The chart included both parents' families and all the adults who supported mother now. The children were all extremely attentive and informative as I kept them all engaged in talking about the different people on the chart and how they supported mother and themselves.

I found it a bit strange making such a practical illustration of mother's support system, but I realized that making the chart was really a form of a good interpretation to all the children. The chart was particularly good for the younger children for it made clear to them in many ways that they didn't need to be a substitute for daddy and thus blur the generational boundaries.

While making the 'family friends chart' I gave three messages to the family:
1. Mother had her adult friends to support her. I encouraged mother to discuss and face her pain in being alone and her need for friends.
2. The children did not need to be mother's companion.
3. Mother, dad and family friends were available to help with their feelings and dad would see them on a regular basis.

Using the family tree

I used the family tree to show how the identified patient may carry the mother's unmet needs from the previous generation. In one session I sat on the floor again with the children and helped the three oldest children to draw part of the family tree. I asked them to find out the information that they didn't know from their mother. They filled in characteristics of various family members and then we tried to discover what happened to their parents when they were aged six, the age of Jack, the boy with night terrors. I also tried to see if the identified patient's position, Jack being the youngest boy, in some way linked with the parent's position in their family of origin.

> While mother and Shirley were talking about how they always got into rows, Shirley, aged three, came to sit next to mother. Then Jack, aged six, came and sat beside mother and she immediately wrapped her arm round his shoulder and smiled. This provided an immense contrast to her other side, where Shirley sat: mother had her arm tightly pressed to her side. I pointed out the position of arm around her son and closed arm to her daughter. I wondered how mother might in some way be linked with an experience she had at Shirley's age. Mother immediately said she had a terrible relationship with her mother. Her mother often neglected her because she was preoccupied with a handicapped child in the family. Mother went on to add that one reason she found it difficult to discipline the children was that she was afraid she would turn out like the maternal grandmother, whom mother experienced as cruel and uncaring. This hostility to her own mother prevented mother from identifying with her mother's helpful parental functions.

Mother's feelings of love intertwined with anger led her to provide cuddles instead of discipline or containment of Shirley's anxiety. Shirley had become an estranged child, holding mother's childhood feelings of being lonely and isolated from her own mother.

Acknowledging the therapist's role as an emotional lifeboat for the family and fears of loss of the therapy

After some time, the family members had each increased their capacity to deal with emotional conflicts and the problem of the parental divorce. They less frequently resorted to their usual defences of denial through cuddling, fighting among the children and giggling at crucial emotionally laden moments in the session. At the time we embarked on a discussion about ending therapy, the children were busily drawing.

> Shirley drew a girl trying to hold onto a lifeboat. The girl was shouting help! There were sharks in the water.

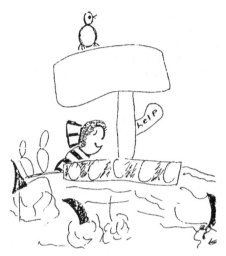

Figure 4.6 Girl holding onto lifeboat: drawing by Shirley.

Earlier in the therapy I had worked extensively on the family's sense of hostility, loss and pain of separation from the therapist between the sessions and during the holidays. I explored the meaning of the drawing with the family and realized that I needed to continue to work for some time longer with the family's anxieties about losing me, their emotional lifeboat.

Helping parents relate to children's play, dreams and drawings

We embarked on the last phase of therapy in which mother was combining her use of parental authority and nurturance with the children. I could see signs that she had internalized experiences of being with me when I had been attentive, thoughtful and responsive to the non-verbalized emotional expressions of the family. However, in the final sessions of therapy, there was a recurrence of the problem.

> Mother complained that now her youngest child, Kismet, three, was waking her at night, coming into her bed and wetting it. I was struck by how the sleep difficulty emerged at the time the family was about to lose me as a support. I remarked on how mother was tempted to cuddle Kismet in bed at night. I linked these activities with the feelings everyone had of being left by dad, husband and now by me.

Subsequently Shirley, aged eight, recounted a recurrent nightmare that she used to have of being left all alone in a pram, abandoned outside a lift. Mother and the four children all discussed their feelings about ending therapy. Kismet said she was tired because her head was 'filled with dreams'. I encouraged mother and Kismet to talk about these dreams each day and to make drawing of anything which bothered Kismet. I suggested that mother tell Kismet that she was there now to help her with the 'frightening monster' about which Kismet complained, but she would not sleep with her at night. Mother was very keen to do this. After two weeks, she reported, with surprise, that Kismet had stopped wetting the bed and wakening at night. Kismet had told her mother of some nightmares and her fear of being eaten by a boy at school.

I described how Kismet's improvement was linked with the family's ability to bear their anxiety in separating from me. I also encouraged the children in the future to feel free to show their drawings to their mother or tell her of any dreams that bothered them. I encouraged mother to imagine and be attentive and receptive to worries that initially were not put into words, but just enter into the drama of their dreams and drawings.

Ultimately it is the parents who must continue providing the emotional understanding necessary for the children to develop in a healthy manner. For this reason, I was keen to express my trust in mother as the person able to foster richness in the expression of intimate feelings in the family. The children had lost their fear that self-expression of feelings of anger or ambivalence were solely bad and would necessarily lead to loss of love. Slowly, with the help of their parents and myself, they were able to repair the 'crack' in their lifeboat which lead to insecurity in the family. Love for each other and a sense of well-being were expressed in David's picture, drawn for his mother at the end of therapy.

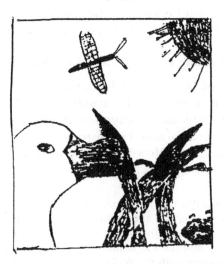

Figure 4.7 A bird eating a plant and resting under the sun: drawing by David.

Summary of my family therapy technique: structured spontaneity in the play arena

The trend in family therapy has often been towards reliance on the verbal contributions of family members. However, young children are a very rich spring from which can come the family's preverbal experiences, pressing for access to consciousness during the session. The children provide access to the unconscious spontaneous healing forces in the family.

My linking child psychotherapy with family therapy, with John's encouragement, led me to use 'structured spontaneity in the play arena' as a primary mode of approach to families with young children. This technique is designed to foster an appreciation of children's play and dreams as a means to express and work on the family's preoccupations, conflicts and phantasies. Often children, particularly when very young, cannot answer direct questions because they do not consciously have the kind of thoughts fitted to giving answers to adult's questions. They have not yet put a name to some of their feelings or their experiences of family life. The children's free play can, however, serve as a commentary on the ongoing relationship between the therapist and the family members. Free play can also serve the same function as the parents' conversation. A very vital contribution can be made by the younger members of the family, if only we allow the children to exist freely in the session, follow their movements and give value and meaning to their non-verbal contributions.

In this family where night terrors existed, I did not ask the children to play, nor did I designate the theme of their play or drawing. Each activity of the children was used by me not as a comment on the inner world experiences of a particular child, but rather as the child's comment to elucidate the family's ongoing external pattern of relationship and the fantasies connected with their internalized family relationships. Through my presence the children were able to bring into their drawings the terror, hostility and love which the family felt. I fostered a dialogue between the child and the image of feelings, which could be pictured and not yet spoken about by the family. I engaged with each of the children and allowed them to spontaneously play and converse with each other and their parents. I provided understanding of the primary feelings and anxieties portrayed, rather than constantly pressing the children for verbal answers to questions. Through this 'structured spontaneity' of the family therapy sessions, the children were gradually able to begin to talk about their terrifying fears, feel the tears under their smiling faces and develop more security in having the unmanageable terrifying experiences known about, deeply faced and contained by themselves and their mother. The night-terrors disappeared within six sessions.

Conclusion

My work with four night-terror families enabled me to notice that the index patient was not permitted to be a child and to pursue and gain mastery over his interests with other children and at school. Instead, out of loyalty and insecure attachment to his parents, he felt paralysed with the burden of attempting to carry out inappropriate roles such as being a parent in the family or quasi-sexual partner to one of the parents. Night terrors resulted, with the child being emotionally needed by the parents, whose marital relationship was fraught with disappointment, anger and despair. The parents had turned to the child as a new source of emotional satisfaction. Their pairing with the child was also an attempt to ward off their psychic pain regarding past lost relationships with their own parents and their own emotional separation (Boszormenyi-Nagy Spark, 1973).

Through family therapy which involved particular attention to spontaneous play and drawing of the children, the family members were enabled to feel emotionally secure enough to face their frustrations rather than evade them. The index patient was thus freed from the paralysing terror of trying to live a lie that he was grown up when in truth he was only a child. The night terrors thus were diminished.

In this process of working with the families, as already mentioned, John Byng-Hall's supportive presence functioned as a bridge for me between child psychoanalytic psychotherapy and family therapy. With the 'bug in my ear', I was helping the family experiencing night-terrors work through their difficulties. I was also having to work through my own anxieties about change and loss of professional identity. It was difficult to incorporate the ideas in John's approaches to family therapy, which differed from those in psychoanalytic psychotherapy. I would become 'unacceptable' to some who felt I should toe the party-line. I would never make a 'traditional family therapist' – whether it be systemic, structural or psychodynamic. What I learned most from John's example was the courage to let go of the accepted beliefs connected with one's own professional cliché;, while searching for what seemed therapeutically useful, both for myself in working with a family and for the family members themselves. For this freedom to use all of me – my Americanness, my child psychotherapy hat, my wish to be more emotionally expressive and dramatic, for this freedom to be me – I have John to thank as a model and as a facilitating presence, as I trained to be a family therapist.

Jeanne Magagna is a child, adult and family psychotherapist heading Psychotherapy Services at Great Ormond Street Hospital for Children, in London. She also works as joint co-ordinator of the child psychotherapy trainings in Centro Studi Martha Harris in Florence and Venice. Her special interests include psychotherapy with children having eating disorders, hallucinations in children and group work for parents and nurses.

Chapter 5
Following a different script in the surgery: working as a systemic psychotherapist in general practice

SARA BARRATT

I have been working as a systemic psychotherapist in a village-based general practice in Hertfordshire since 1988. About 25 per cent of the referrals from GPs involve couples or families, the remainder being made up equally of men and women who may bring partners for the occasional appointment. Some people return to see me from time to time as crises occur, or I may come across them in the waiting room or hear of them from their GPs. I see myself as a member of a multidisciplinary team in the surgery and work closely with the doctors when there are patients about whom we share concerns. I seek a patient's permission to talk to the their GP about our work and only once has this been refused. Most people are pleased and reassured that we work collaboratively with them.

This chapter is about my work in general practice and the influence of John Byng-Hall's ideas on my thinking and approach. Family scripts play an important part in our responses to illness. Our ideas about health and illness are embedded in the experiences of our families of origin and our cultural beliefs. While the GP is the first port of call when we are ill, the surgery can also be an important focal point for a local community. It is central to our lives at significant times, such as the birth of children or when there is serious or chronic illness. In some communities it is a meeting place for neighbours and groups.

Before making a referral to a counsellor or therapist, the GP may work with the patient to look at the range of interventions available, and so introduce the idea of psychological rather biomedical help. The patient may have distressing physical symptoms and feel misunderstood if the GP's focus is on the psychosomatic and suggests that they may be helped through psychotherapy. Patients with symptoms such as chronic pain or headaches sometimes feel that such a referral means that the GP does not believe the pain to be 'real'. We often find that it is helpful for the GP and psychotherapist to work together with the patient to find ways of treating both the physical and emotional aspects of the pain. Some patients who are under emotional pressure and stress also face a powerful cultural injunction against mental illness that means it is only possible to represent their distress by talking about physical symptoms. In some families, where the dominant discourse is to equate illness with weakness, it often difficult for a member to consult a doctor about any symptoms, particularly if they may be viewed as having a psychological origin.

Constructing my script

When I first read about John Byng-Hall's ideas about family scripts, I felt that they were more appropriate to people from traditional cultures where there is a strong sense of family. My own disconnection from parts of my parents' family history meant that my awareness of such scripts was severely limited, either to repair or replicate (Rolland, 1994). I had to invent traditions in my family of procreation and we have established a number of rituals which have been built up as our own family traditions.

In trying to make sense of my past I have tried to construct a coherent story from the snippets of memory and the few stories that I have been told. I was nine years old and living with a foster family when my mother died. I had not seen her for several months and by the time I was told of her death her funeral had already taken place. My father, when I saw him, made it clear he did not want to talk about her. This denial persisted throughout his life, though pieces of information occasionally slipped out. His response may have grown out of a very British post-war injunction against talking about painful experiences. As my mother had no immediate living relatives it was difficult for me to gather the jigsaw about her family life together, particularly as I was living away from home. Any information gathered from neighbours or friends was therefore very valuable.

I have sometimes wondered, however, if I imagined some of the events that I apparently recall and the confirmation of my memories through discussions with others has been very helpful in validating my experiences. For example, a school friend with whom I have recently reconnected after some 30 years remembers the difficulties I had with my father and his attempts to help me to escape from the family. Until I met him I had thought that I had been a particularly difficult young person but, listening to his recollection of my father's refusal to communicate with me, sometimes for weeks at a time, my behaviour made sense.

I wonder how it is, for those who have had the opposite experience, who have immediate access to their family history. They have so much information to process, and the dilemma of reconciling their memories with a diversity of stories of which there may be many versions which form the totality of the family discourse.

With the increase in social mobility, many of us no longer live in settled communities. Since the Second World War Britain has seen huge changes in its patterns of migration. For some families this is a choice driven by work demands or unemployment, while for others political changes or social tragedies have necessitated a move away from their place of origin. This often leads to a continued yearning for roots – the place and community where we grew up. No doubt John Byng-Hall's departure from his birthplace, Kenya, contributed to a greater interest in family of origin issues – settling in London he was separated from his childhood both by physical distance and by the development of polio that changed his hopes for his life (Byng-Hall, 1995b). From my reading of aspects of his life, I see him as someone who has found ways to overcome the limitations that his body tries to present to him.

General practice: confidentiality

When a patient is referred to me, I make it clear that I work with the team and feed back the themes of our work and any concern I might have to the referring GP. GPs usually see individuals and confidentiality as of primary importance; as a systemic psychotherapist I am accustomed to working with families and to include different family members in the work. When a young man was referred to me with sexual problems and started talking about his father I realized that I had worked with the latter a few years previously. The father had been referred because of impotence and some of the family patterns began to fall into place. The young man was unaware that I had seen his father and I found it difficult to set aside some of the things I knew about the family. When discussing this difficulty with the GP who had referred both father and son, the differences in our professional scripts became apparent: for GP's connecting symptoms manifested in different family members could be constructed as a breach of confidentiality, for a systemic practitioner this cross-generational occurrence generated important treatment hypotheses.

The family stories that we are told about sickness usually affect our view of ourselves and our capacity to cope with ill-health (Greenhalgh and Hurwitz, 1998). For example, when we feel ill statements such as 'you always did make a fuss when you weren't well' may be profoundly inhibiting. As a therapist in general practice the moment one sees the patient's eyes light up is when making a comment that validates an experience as painful or difficult which others close to the patient discount or disqualify.

James, aged 34, came to see me with symptoms of anxiety that were paralysing him at work as an electrical engineer. He was worried that he was wasting my time as there were 'people with more serious problems than me'. James's fear that he might make a mistake led to a series of worries, which taken to their conclusion, for example, would lead to the flooding of the city of London because he may have forgotten to turn off a switch. He would often return to work at weekends on some pretext in order to check that he had turned off all the switches and locked all the doors.

He was the eldest child of the family, with two younger sisters. In describing some of the patterns in his family of origin, he spoke of living in constant fear as he and his sisters would be beaten for any mistake they made, such as breaking a glass or spilling something on the floor. He felt disloyal to his family in talking about these childhood experiences that he had never considered abusive. As an adult he lived in constant fear of being found out for committing some unknown misdemeanour. He was in a sexual relationship with Julia who continually criticized him for failing to dress or behave appropriately, and who sought to control him. She was married but said that she would leave her husband when James treated her better. It was difficult to understand how James would consider acquiescing to such demands; my response would have been to leave, but I recognized that he did not perceive this as an option. I worked hard to understand his script that challenge leads to abuse and we worked on ways in which he could start to recognize what he wanted and to think particularly about what he would want in a relationship – he was not ready to act. We started by working on ways in which he could negotiate better with his boss at work and with his parents. In time James found ways of disagreeing with his parents. He has now ended his relationship with Julia and is beginning to initiate relationships with other people and assert himself more at work. He describes feeling able to relax in a way that he has never done before.

People I have worked with who have experienced strong criticism or abuse in their families of origin have find it unthinkable to challenge their parents for fear that disagreement will lead to a complete breakdown in the relationship. They are often surprised that by changing the way they position themselves with their families of origin they can free themselves from the constraining family script and become more confident. As with many abusive relationships, there is an idea that talking about distressing events from the past will be catastrophic. Clients are often surprised that both they and their families are relieved when change starts. For example,

James was frightened that if he talked to his parents, particularly his father, about their behaviour during his childhood, they would accuse him of lying and there would be an estrangement in the relationship. Instead, we worked on ways he could start to challenge his father in order to feel less frightened of him, through disagreeing with his father's racist statements that he found intolerable. In challenging such statements, he has found that in time his father has changed the way he talks and abandoned racist comments. Seeing this success emboldened James to raise some of the past abusive events that were still upsetting him. His father has started to respond more respectfully towards him. James has now adopted these techniques in work and in his personal relationships and is beginning to rewrite his script. He now describes himself as someone who is in charge of his life, confident and competent, and who can take risks without panicking. When I showed James the extract for this chapter he said that it helped him to realize how far he had come.

Family scripts and the unknown

The GP holds the coherent story of our medical lives from birth to death. As one with a limited family history, strangely the only place where some knowledge of my early years is lodged is in my medical records! This means that a stranger has access to more information about me than I have. My childhood memories are punctuated by dramatic images of illness that I can neither explain nor have ever considered asking my GP about. Why do I remember standing on the kitchen table screaming, with a nurse about to do something to me – why am I terrified of injections? Why do I have large scars from what looks like needles? I will probably never know and writing this chapter has stimulated these latent memories.

I have worked with a number of families and individuals who have adopted children or who have been adopted. For adoptees the absence of information can be particularly difficult especially when needing to know about family health. Simple questions as to whether there any allergies in your family or history of high blood pressure can cause distress. Parents who initially hope that they will tell their adopted children all they know about their birth families, may find it hard to answer such questions and it is often hard for children to ask. Sometimes this is for fear of causing unnecessary distress but, paradoxically, the absence of such conversations also leads to a gulf between parents and children.

Susan talked to me about how awkward she felt when she was pregnant and could not answer questions about her mother's medical history or pregnancy. Such questions at a time when women may be thinking about their own origins can be unsettling and can sometimes act as a trigger in an attempt to trace birth families. Helping clients to decide whether to trace families of origin and whether to discuss such a decision with adoptive families makes me aware of how complex these decisions are.

The wish to trace birth families, which in general practice may start with a wish to trace medical history, is like leaping with someone into the unknown. To embark on such a journey is both exciting and frightening. I am always aware of the ways clients are going to manage the new information or its absence (what can never be known) and feel very privileged to be able to share the joys and disappointments of discovery. John Byng-Hall (1995a) is influenced heavily by Bowlby's (1988) ideas about attachment theory and the importance of a secure base for children. For adopted children attachment has inevitably been difficult. In general practice, I am readily contacted by patients who have been adopted and who are beginning to seek their birth parents. In this context, I always seek to provide a secure and accessible base.

Susan had been referred by her GP because she had a history of undiagnosed physical symptoms. She welcomed the idea of talking about her relationship with her partner whom she saw as unsympathetic. She has a small child who is asthmatic and this had triggered her decision to trace her birth family; she had made the request for her original birth certificate at the time of referral to me. We had talked about what she hoped for in looking for her birth parents but she was devastated when her birth certificate came back with the address of her birth as a large 'subnormality' hospital. Her idealized hopes for a glorious reunion were shattered but she continued the search and found her birth mother who had been hospitalized as a 'moral defective', i.e. a woman who was unmarried and pregnant in the 1950s. Susan learned that her mother had been discharged at the time when 'care in the community' was the emphasis of social policy and found her whereabouts. She was able to fill in some of the gaps in her life story but decided that she did not have the emotional resources to meet her birth mother's needs and therefore only kept a tenuous connection. Susan advertised in a national newspaper and found a sister with whom she was able to develop a relationship. During this time I worked with her, supporting her processing this new information and identifying what she wanted for herself through it. She continued to visit her adoptive mother and faced the struggle of telling her about her search for her birthparents. My task then became to help her reflect on the emerging relationships with different family members and through providing a 'secure base' from which she could work to integrate the different strands in her family experience.

Susan's preoccupation with this work led to tensions with her partner. He was many years older and felt set aside by Susan's interest in her birth family. Her partner joined the sessions in which they worked on the readjustment of their relationship, while Susan continued to negotiate her relationship with her adoptive mother and her birth sister. Her understanding of her roots from a medical and emotional perspective were important to her as a parent in establishing her family of procreation.

Diagnosis and general practice

We visit the doctor with a specific symptom and meet for a limited length of time. The traditional consultation is one in which the patient describes the symptom and the doctor makes a diagnosis and prescribes treatment. Asking for information on our medical records, though a right, is still for many to step outside the rules and traditions of such a relationship.

Traditionally the GP group practice has been one in which medical colleagues can expect to work together throughout their professional lives. Each may take a different role, in a way which reflects the division and resources within the family. Patients visit different GPs with different symptoms – one practice partner may be better at listening to distressing accounts of what is happening in a patient's lives while another may be good at providing a quick diagnosis and prescribing medication. From my perspective as a systemic psychotherapist I can often guess the referring GP by the nature of the patient's declared problem, thus different team members attract patients with certain types of problems or are more responsive to therapeutic need.

When the patient's description of the symptoms do not make it possible to make a clear diagnosis, or the symptoms do not respond as expected to medication, a GP, who is systemically aware, may start to ask about the family stories about the symptoms and beliefs about illness, and the response to the symptoms of those close to the patient. When we go to the doctor we have about seven minutes to describe our symptoms. Inevitably patients become more anxious when the GP asks questions about current relationships in the family or about our family of origin. Such interest is unexpected and paradoxically may give rise to the fear that the diagnosis must be serious for the GP to show such interest!

As previously stated, the pressures we have, through work or relationships, affect our physical and mental health (Asen and Tomson, 1987). For many families health and illness are also connected to poverty and unemployment. Jim and Dorothy, a couple in their fifties were frequent attenders at the surgery in Sheffield where I work with the GP, Jack Czauderna. The surgery is in an area of high unemployment and provides services for a large, multicultural community. Jim and Dorothy visited the GP approximately twice a month. Dorothy had suffered serious depression over the years that required hospitalisation. Jim had been made redundant from the local steelworks and devoted his time to caring for his wife, on one occasion discharging her from hospital to look after her at home. When Dorothy started to get better and was able to resume her life, Jim became depressed and was prescribed anti-depressant medication. In a joint consultation, Jack and I talked with the couple about the patterns of depression in their lives. It became clear that Jim first became depressed when he was made redundant: he developed serious physical symptoms, chronic pain in his joints and headaches, that he could not account for. Though Dorothy initially said that she was fully recovered from depression and believed she could now spend time at home alone, she later reconsidered and said this would be difficult for her and that she would wish Jim to be with her. He talked about the desolation he felt after the loss of the job which he had held since leaving school. He felt that he could not face the idea of permanent unemployment – his identity was as a steel worker and family provider. It was less shaming to be unable to work because of ill health than because he was unable to find work, he said.

The contexts for our lives affect whether we can allow ourselves to be ill. It is not only the family of origin experience of illness and care, but wider socio-economic pressures which affect the way we respond to illness. Having time off work has a diversity of meanings for different occupational groups as well as the family history of illness and treatment. The denial of the significance of the illness may mean that people continue to drive themselves and to convince themselves that they are well because the alternative is to acknowledge their fear of diminishing health or aging. In some families illness is a time to be looked after and comforted; in others, it is a time when there is little attention or caregiving, which compound the feeling of being unwell. For example, some children may visit the GP and take a week off school with sore throats, while others with the same symptoms may be told to stop making a fuss.

Transgenerational beliefs about illness

In families in which there is a history of specific illnesses, it may be difficult to believe that new generations will outlive their parents'. Transgenerational ideas about illness and family events punctuate the life-cycle and may create a health or death crisis either for a family member or a family relationship. Approaching the age when a parent or grandparent was seriously or terminally ill can be a time of anxiety. These are sometimes described as the 'time bombs that are embedded in the script'. Such worries often lead to increased protectiveness of children and concern for family members people as they approach the critical age.

Huygen, a Dutch GP, studied 200 families in his practice between 1945 and 1965 (1978); 100 were described as younger, or 'in the expanding and stabilising stage' and 100 were 'in the contracting' stage. He found that the number of nervous disorders increased over the years of marriage. Looking at the transgenerational patterns of illness he discovered that if one parent in a family had many periods of illness it was likely that both the children and the other parent would show the same phenomenon: 'The correlation between parent and children were much greater than between the parents themselves.' He completed genograms of the families to study transgenerational patterns of illness and found diagnoses and patterns of consultation were repeated over the generations. Huygen started to work with family therapists, and found that this approach provided a more useful intervention for the patients who consulted more frequently. These findings are reflected in our practice though the mobility of our catchment population makes it difficult to follow many families through the generations.

Margaret was referred by her GP because she was depressed and anxious; she had not slept for many weeks and he was concerned that she was suicidal. He asked me to see her urgently to decide with her whether she needed hospitalization. She attended the appointment with her husband. Though she had experienced depressive illnesses in the past, she was frightened by her current condition. A combination of circumstances had lead to the distress. Margaret and George have two children aged 19 and 16. Stephen, the younger, had been born with heart problems and had not been expected to survive. After a series of operations he had developed into a robust adolescent. Six months prior to the referral, his closest friend had died suddenly of meningitis. This resurrected Margaret's fears about her son's survival and she described the fear of death that preoccupied her. During our first meeting she recalled that her mother had had a depressive illness when she, Margaret, was 16 and had been expected to give up her own plans to stay at home and care for the family. George's mother was diagnosed with a manic-depressive illness when he was a child. Both felt that they came from families in which women were seen as entirely dependent on men.

The couple had not spoken to Stephen about their distress at his friend's death and felt unable to talk to the boy's family because of their intense feelings, and guilt that they did not have the right to be so upset since their own son was still alive. Margaret worried about her own death, which she links with her mother's illness. A visit to a medium to try and understand this preoccupation accelerated the emotional crisis. The family had a strongly held belief that worries and feelings should not be voiced though they observed one another closely. Margaret checked

Stephen's letters from friends to find out how he felt and, despite retreating to bed for three months, talking to no one, she believed that her son did not know she was unwell.

In our work together we started to discuss the risks involved if the family were to start to talk and listen to one another more seriously. Their communication beliefs and the combination of recent events triggered a depression that reverberated with Margaret's life at 16. Our work focused increasingly on couple work, and as Margaret's health improved – she no longer stayed in bed all day and started to be less dependent on George – he become more anxious and convinced that she would leave him. They recognise the patterns in their families of origin and Margaret is struggling to find ways of maintaining her new feeling of autonomy while reassuring her partner that she is committed to their relationship.

Physical illness

Physical illness affects all of us. 'From childhood onwards our personal and family experiences of illness shape us a surely as the food we eat and the love or rejection we experience' (McDaniels et al., 1997). They maintain that therapists should be aware of the way their own experiences of illness have shaped their lives and their relationships with patients. Such experiences influence our beliefs and decisions about whether it is better to suffer in silence or to seek treatment immediately from the 'illness expert'. As therapists, we are more familiar with working with the psychological rather than the physical effects of illness and we may overlook the distress caused by physical symptoms or to take account of its impact. Margaret had been brought up to discount her feelings and to believe that she had a responsibility to 'parent' her parents. This is a familiar pattern for people I see in general practice who suffer an acute and serious depression.

John, aged 54, was referred by his GP with depression. Like Margaret, he believed that personal duty to family was important. He had been made redundant six months earlier from a managerial job in a firm in which he had worked since leaving college. Although he had anticipated this event, he had made no plans as to how he would manage his time and had persuaded himself that it would not effect him. On finishing work he set up projects to keep himself busy and worked harder than ever, not sleeping and losing contact with his close friends from work. A car accident, for which he was responsible, left him suicidal and unable to cope.

Our work addressed John's experiences of physical illness in childhood (Kleinman, 1988). He had attended school for about half time, spending the remainder of the time in hospital or at home with his disabled father who was emotionally abusive to him. He suffered humiliation at home and at school. As soon as he left home he would not 'allow himself to be ill' though he contracted TB and later had surgery for a serious back problem – he returned to work before doctors said he was physically ready. He drove himself to succeed and thought the appropriate response to any setback was to work harder. The redundancy had left him unable to apply this strategy and his tendency to avoid emotions meant that he had not recognized his own sadness or depression.

He characterized himself as the bad person in the family. The youngest of three brothers he was seen as a failure as he had not achieved academically. During our work he started to rewrite this description of himself. His older brother had been imprisoned for fraud and John had had to bail him out, while his other brother had entirely cut himself off from the family in contrast to John who had provided a home for his mother and financial support in the years up to her death. It was difficult for him to reconcile the family description of him with this account of him as a kind and supportive son and brother. He had worked hard to be 'good enough' but felt he had always failed. The rewriting of this script was essential in helping John to start to see himself differently and to take less responsibility for compensating his brothers for their own difficulties.

Culture and health

For many families in a multicultural society, Western medical interventions can create tensions and misunderstandings with the inherent danger of a complete breakdown in communication (Al-Issa, 1995). Anne Fadiman's book, *The Spirit Catches You and You Fall Down*, gives a moving account of the tragedy of a Hmong refugee family living in America. (The Hmong people come from north-west Laos; 150,000 people fled the country after the communist coup in 1975.) Their child, Lia, developed epilepsy, for which the Hmong explanation is 'the spirit catches you and you fall down'. In their culture an epileptic child is a special child. Fadiman demonstrates how the collision of the American and Hmong cultures led to a communication breakdown. The American doctors had strong beliefs about the medical needs of Lia, who had her first fit when she was three months old. The family's way of healing was at odds with that of the American health system and this led to a court order placing Lia in foster care. The book demonstrates the tragedy of misunderstanding in which the dominant culture used its power to dictate medical intervention at odds with the family culture. In such situations, 'professional healers' have to work hard to give up some of their long held beliefs to meet the needs of their patients.

I was asked to consult to a group of health workers in Singapore who wanted advice on how to manage a patient who was resistant to treatment. The patient was a young Chinese woman with two small children who had been diagnosed with cancer. The workers were concerned that she would die if she did not agree to surgery and chemotherapy. The woman lived with her husband and his family, who used traditional Chinese methods of healing and had sent her to a healer. Her employer had suggested that she attend the hospital which used Western medical interventions. During the course of the consultation it became clear to the workers that the young woman would have no family support or child care if she accepted their treatment and would be isolated from her culture. They accepted that the best option for her was to take the treatment supported by her family and saw their task to support her in whatever decision she made.

Psychosomatic illness: shame

Traditional western medicine divides interventions between physical and psychological, often divorcing the two. Thus, when a patient attends the GP with symptoms which need further investigation, a choice has to be made between interventions for the mind or body. Our system does not offer a 'both/and' possibility. For the patient who believes his headaches are physical in origin, a referral to a specialist who works with emotional problems could lead to a breakdown in the relationship with the doctor. As we have seen, where a GP and therapist are able to work together, the medical and the emotional, 'body and mind', can be discussed in the consultation.

Reg attended the surgery with chronic back pain; he had been unable to work for several months. The GP was also treating his wife for depression. Reg wanted to talk about the current medication that was not working. He had always been fit, indeed the strongest person in the gym, but now, at 55, he felt that his body was letting him down and he'd noticed that younger people were doing better than he. While he could talk to the GP about his pain, as a therapist I was able to explore about his pain at growing older and being overtaken by younger people. The gym was an important escape from his wife and he left the consultation thinking about how he could reduce his activity in the gym to save his back while talking to his wife about activities they could share. At the next consultation, two weeks later, Reg reported that he had worked hard to change his priorities and that things were much better.

Tom was referred because he had been consulting his GP weekly. He suffered from sickness and headaches for two years since his wife had told him that she had just finished an affair with a work colleague. Tom did not feel that his problem could be helped by therapy but he'd agreed to see me to 'shut Dr Smith up'. Our work then focused on what would need to change for Dr Smith to feel happier. We agreed to meet for four sessions, two of which included Tom's wife. The couple worked on the issue of trust. Tom came with the belief that his wife had to prove that she was trustworthy, although he had no idea how she could demonstrate this. The balance changed to one where Tom needed to work on his ability to trust. Their conjoint work changed the way they related to one another. The symptoms mysteriously disappeared and Tom was left wondering what he would do without the symptoms! This was the next issue to be examined. The outcome, of course, was that Dr Smith was happier, particularly as Tom's consultations reduced in frequency.

Depression in general practice

The majority of referrals to a therapist in general practice come under the broad category of 'depression'. Research (Boyd and Weissman, 1982) has shown that 13–20 per cent of us can expect to suffer from depressive symptoms at some stage in our lives, while 5.8 per cent (Regier et al., 1988) will suffer from a major depression. The general practice research database (National Statistics, 2000) gives an analysis of patient treatments between 1994 and 1998. It shows that approximately 26 male and 66 female patients per thousand were treated for depression and that 22 male and 53 female patients per thousand were treated for anxiety. In this study medication was the treatment provided.

While the accepted alternative treatment to medication for depression is cognitive behavioural therapy (CBT), recent research (Leff et al., 2000) shows that systemic psychotherapy which includes a partner is more successful. In describing their work on this project, Elsa Jones and Eia Asen (2000) have shown that the outcome is better than drugs or CBT. They report that 50 per cent of depressed patients in the study had experienced sexual abuse in childhood and around 40 per cent reported abuse in their relationship with a current partner. In my experience in general practice, where patients are referred without diagnosis, I find that at least 30 per cent of women have been sexually abused and approximately 20 per cent of men. At least 50 per cent of all clients have been the victims of ongoing physical abuse during childhood.

Although referred with various symptoms, all the patients mentioned in this chapter described themselves as suffering from depression, which manifested itself in different ways. Some were willing to invite their partners to the sessions. The GP, unlike the therapist, knows the patient over many years and can observe patterns of consultation and are in a better position to identify the latent depression. In addition to including other family members in my work where possible, I am also able to work closely with the GP when a patient is at the critical stage of depression.

When John (described above) was referred, he was seriously suicidal and saw this as his only option. He had a court case pending for the car accident, he felt useless at home where he was behaving tyrannically and had noticed that his children and partner were avoiding him wherever possible. He considered taking an overdose of tablets or deliberately crashing the car. In our work with John, I phoned him twice during the week and he had weekly appointments with the GP and with me. This continued for 2–3 weeks until he began to feel safe. While he did not want to include his partner in our work, he agreed to my talking to her on the telephone. She found that this helped her to cope in the difficult times they were having. When further crises arose, the GP again joined us briefly in our sessions. John said this helped him to feel safer and thought our approach was important to his recovery.

In working with depressed patients in crisis, my GP colleagues and I have found that by working closely together we have been better able to keep our patients safe during the critical stages. We often take the first part of our initial session to meet the patient together. If the GP and patient feel that medication is appropriate, this is discussed and weekly consultations with the GP and me are arranged. It is made clear that this is our practice and at critical stages I telephone patients between sessions.

Sexuality

The therapist in a general practice may be the first person with whom we can talk about sexuality. Patients referred with a diagnosis of depression usually start to talk about their sexual relationships that have felt uncomfortable. In a predominantly white, rural area, there is little opportunity to talk about difference, whether cultural or sexual. It is important for the therapist in general practice to initiate discussion of sex and sexuality. In my experience people who live in a heterosexual culture have little opportunity to explore their sexuality in their friendship groups, particularly if they think they may be gay or lesbian. Many people have rigid family beliefs about sexuality that exclude the possibility that a family member might be gay. This becomes paralysing for everyone.

More than 25 per cent of my current surgery patients were referred for depression, which is related to concerns about sexuality. For men this has been mainly about seeking out prostitutes for sexual experiences unacceptable in their marriages; for women it has been the exploration of the possibility they might be lesbians and the risk involved in testing this through experience.

For a married woman the decision to develop a lesbian relationship is accompanied by a concern about it breaking up her marriage; for single women the prejudice of the family of origin can be disabling. Jane, aged 28, was referred for depression and, after several sessions in which we discussed her previous, violent, heterosexual relationship, I wondered aloud if she had ever considered that she might be gay. After initial consternation, she started to feel relieved and this helped her to understand some of the feelings she was experiencing. We worked together for over a year in which she examined the beliefs about sexuality in her family of origin and friendship group. She also started to take the adventurous risk of exploring new sexual relationships. In time Jane was able to talk about her sexuality with her parents and brother and moved into a new lesbian relationship. She was able to rewrite her story and gain the support of her family of origin and also discovered that her uncle was gay. Jane began to visit him and his partner, who helped her to manage the changes involved in moving between rural Hertfordshire and the gay scene in London. She recently wrote to say that she was settled in a relationship, though thought her partner needed to do some work with her family of origin.

It is important for the therapist to initiate a conversation about sex and sexual relationships. If we fail to, patients may believe that it is because we cannot help them in this area of their lives. Confidentiality especially needs to be negotiated. When someone begins to talk about sexual issues, they need to be assured that the feedback to the GP is discussed with them and that they approve of what information is given. Failure to clarify this may lead to a serious breakdown of trust.

Conclusion

Working in general practice is an exciting process of being able to work within a community and have the possibility of providing long-term spells of brief therapy. General practice is unique in providing a service for patients over their life span, and does not restrict its response to categories or ages. The surgery is a familiar place, local and accessible. If patients are not defined too rigidly as having particular health needs – either psychological or physical – they are more willing to attend. Patients are referred because of a range of difficulties which often originate in crises at work or in family relationships. The relationship that the GP has with patients over time leads to a continuity and a recognition of patterns that are strongly related to family scripts. As a systemic psychotherapist, my participation may be a beneficial intervention in the GP–patient relationship which helps to explore the impact of family scripts and can have a long-lasting impact.

Through being part of the community, we are aware of aspects of patients' lives that are not discussed in the therapeutic relationship. As with Admiral Byng, John Byng-Hall's eminent ancestor (Byng-Hall, 1982a), we know, for instance, that a patient' s grandfather was a local politician involved in a corruption scandal, and that this will have an affect the way the community views his children and grandchildren. We may also know about secret relationships and fears that help us understand symptoms, although we cannot talk about them in the session. Ideas of family script have led me to view general practice as a secure base that gives the GP, therapist, patient and family the opportunity to work together in rescripting the experiences.

I would like to thank the people I have worked with in general practice and the patients I have seen who have read these accounts and added their views. I would particularly like to mention Jack Czauderna in Sheffield and the Nap Surgery in Kings Langley, Hertfordshire for providing great opportunities for collaborative practice.

Sara Barratt trained as a social worker and worked for Hertfordshire County Council, specializing in child protection, fostering and adoption. She completed her training in family therapy at the Tavistock Clinic. From 1989 to 1999 her work included family therapy with the South Bucks Health Authority adult psychiatric services. Since 1988 she has worked in general practice as a therapist and a consultant to GPs, was Director of Training at the Institute of Family Therapy (1994–6) and is currently a member of the systems team at the Tavistock Clinic, where she co-organizes the Masters course in Systemic Psychotherapy. She is a member of the Childhood Depression Research Project and of the Fostering and Adoption team.

Chapter 6
The theatre, the family and the scripted world

Kate Daniels

Augusto Boal, Brazilian theatre director and director of Centre of Theatre of the Oppressed, tells an ancient Chinese fable about how theatre was discovered: the story concerns Xua-Xua who lived hundreds of thousands of years ago in pre-human, pre-language times. Having given birth to a child she believed it to be a tiny part of her body. At times, as it grew older it seemed to be a very disobedient part of her body. One day she looked for her small body and could not find it because it had gone off with the pre-human man, Li-Peng, its father. She cried because she had lost part of herself and she wanted to get her baby-body back. When she found it, she was upset that it refused to obey her and stay with her. This refusal forced her to realise that her baby-body was somebody else with its own needs and desires. They were two separate people. This recognition helped her to identify herself and ask questions of herself. Who was she? Who was her child? Where were they? What would happen next time if her belly swelled up? Xua-Xua looked for the answers by looking at herself and asking these questions and that is when she became human.

> In this moment theatre was discovered . . . At that moment she was at one and the same time Actor and Spectator. She was Spectactor. In discovering theatre the being became human. This is theatre. The art of looking at ourselves. (Boal, 1992)

The Chinese fable is not concerned with oedipal interpretations, structural notions of enmeshment or ideas of 'leaving home', although all of these might be extracted from the story. Its interest is in the new and curious eyes with which an experience is observed and a narrative created and it is in that process that theatre and therapy find their first meeting place.

This chapter is about that meeting place. It is about John Byng-Hall's notion of the 'shared metaphor' of scripts, a metaphor which immediately

123

invites us to take a lateral jump into other scripts – the world of plays and films. It explores some of the conjunctions between the family scripts in the play text and the family scripts that John Byng-Hall discusses in his book *Rewriting Family Scripts*. It is about how we look at ourselves, using the medium of formal theatre.

When I began my family therapy training at the Family Institute in Cardiff in 1980 I had a background in theatre and was familiar with the well-established models of psychodrama and drama therapy (Jones, 1996; Moreno, 1946, 1959; Williams, 1989) and the rich contribution these models make to therapy. However, I was struck by a particular and different correspondence between systemic family therapy and theatre. This was to do with the way systemic family therapy chose to 'look at' itself in relation to its client group. There was the audience behind the one-way screen, analysing, assessing and experiencing vicariously the drama being played on stage in the therapy room. There were also the actors, therapist included, on the one hand aware of and 'performing' for their audience, and, on the other hand, totally immersed in the drama they were enacting. The whispered hush in the dark of the consulting room was similar to the contained energy and tension that is felt backstage during a performance. The lively discussion afterwards reflected the discharge of this tension among both actors and audience. There were scripts written up for case discussion or publication, and there were the rehearsals – the role plays.

It seemed that by creating the one-way screen, family therapy had begun construction of its own theatre. Lynn Hoffman points to this in her book, *Foundations of Family Therapy*: 'The screen turned psychotherapy into a bicameral interaction ... One had two places to sit. One could take a position, and have somebody else take a position, commenting on or reviewing that position' (Hoffman, 1981). Subsequently, the development of the reflecting team extended this idea and provided family systems work with its own variation of the Greek chorus (Kaftanzi, 1997).

For a number of years after that initial experience, I moved quite literally between two worlds – two 'theatres'. I was job-sharing the setting-up and running of a family therapy/mediation project and at the same time I was acting in summer repertory seasons. I would go from rehearsals for an adaptation of *Cider with Rosie*, Laurie Lee's autobiographical tale about growing up in a family with an absent father, to interviews with separating couples struggling to work out contact arrangements for their children. I was interested in the way these two worlds mirrored each other and I became aware that I was part of the reflection of each. My work as a therapist contributed to my analysis of the various roles I played on stage. Equally my experience as an actor influenced my work as a therapist. This was firstly in thinking about theatre as a *form* which provides a metaphor for therapy – the stage and the audience: the rehearsals and the performance – and secondly, in terms of my experience of the play text itself. The ideas and the language that constitute theatrical form became important tools in my therapist's repertoire. The plays in which I was performing illuminated my understanding of the human relations with which I worked.

These are the areas I want to explore in this chapter in the light of Byng-Hall's work. In the first part I will look at what he calls the 'shared metaphor' and explore the way the vocabulary and ideas of theatre can help us in our thinking about families and therapy. I also want to introduce briefly some of the ideas of playwrights Bertolt Brecht and Dario Fo that connect most vividly with systemic work. In the second part I will investigate the script itself and look at the way family scripts are presented through the lens of the playwright, using examples from Arthur Miller and Anton Chekhov.

Shared metaphor

In using the term 'script' with families, John Byng-Hall was conscious of using a metaphor that can immediately be understood by clients – scripts are, after all, a common feature of our cultural life through television, theatre and film. The idea of a script offers the possibility for other associated metaphors to be developed and used to reconstruct family stories, rewrite family scripts. When we talk about a 'family drama', for example, the word 'drama' connects in our minds with action, conflict or crisis.

The theatre as a general metaphor available to therapists and clients alike has broad scope. It can accommodate different positions and conflicting experiences. One can, for example, be 'on stage', 'sitting in the audience', 'under the spotlight', 'waiting in the wings', 'playing to the gallery' or 'making a scene'. These are all terms in everyday use that capture complex experiences and connect them to powerful images. Children brought to therapy as a 'problem' might well feel that they are under the spotlight. Such an expression implies the presence of an audience watching and though, on the one hand, the child might enjoy being 'centre stage', being under the spotlight puts them under pressure – it is a lonely place and can be uncomfortably hot!

The power of a metaphor depends on the breadth of meaning it carries from one context to another. For example, the verb 'to improvise' means to create something, to extemporize, to make something up spontaneously. However, in order to improvise it is generally accepted that you must feel some confidence and security within yourself, or the setting and the people that provide your context (Byng-Hall, 1995b). Actors are usually given warm-up exercises before they are asked to improvise, and they are trained in improvisation. The more comfortable they are with improvising the more readily they are able to use it as a tool. Improvising is something that families can be helped to learn when they want to explore something new. The rehearsal process offers the opportunity to practice improvisation, and I use the idea of rehearsal regularly in my work, to help family members to think of change as a process that they are allowed to practice and stumble over. In rehearsal they can practice new roles and try out new ways of being – new scripts. As an actor I found rehearsals more fun than performances. Rehearsals are the place where you are part of something new being created. In rehearsals 'getting it right' too early is frowned upon; it is expected that you will go wrong, forget your moves or mess up your lines as you work to develop your character. That development process is vital and requires time and help from colleagues. Actors recognize, early on, how dependent they are on each other and that this interdependence is a helpful and creative thing.

The metaphor of theatre thus offers alternative values to many of the injunctions with which therapists and families struggle in their work and relationships. The adult world is a serious place of hard work and important weighty considerations and in the case of most therapists, working all day with clients, it is a 'problem-saturated' environment. Contrariwise, there is something playful and childlike about the world of the stage. In this world we say 'Let's pretend ...', practice being someone else, dress up and paint our faces and tell stories. We invoke the imaginative and creative impulses and encourage silliness as part of our explorations. When I run theatre workshops for therapists, I am always struck by the sense of release with which participants engage in the action, the play and the creative exercises.

So what of the play itself? How helpful is it for us as therapists to look at ourselves and our work through that lens? A play can be a rich learning tool for any therapist who wants to examine and understand the patterns and processes of human interaction and to have these compressed and displayed before them in a two-hour slot.

With the impact of realism on nineteenth-century theatre, the theatre world began to talk about plays revealing a 'slice of life' and of theatre as the 'fourth wall', as though what audiences were seeing was what really went on in people's homes. But plays are not real mirrors. Plays are a vision or a slice of life that has been refashioned. They are compositions that conform to certain artistic imperatives. The slice of life one sees on stage is far removed from the day-to-day, humdrum human interaction. Teaching playwriting to university drama students I sent them off to write out five minutes of overheard conversation and then to refashion it to make it script-worthy. They were amazed at how little of the conversation was of any value for a stage play; so much of what they recorded was aimless chit-chat. It is the reconstructing of life stories using the artistic conventions of storytelling for the stage – the dramaturgy – that makes plays a useful learning tool for the therapist. To 'tell' a story well, a playwright must construct it in a particular way using particular devices: the juxtaposing of images and characters or the manipulation of space, time and language – the use of symbols. In this way the complex mechanics of human interaction are revealed and a play becomes a fascinating family case study. *Death of a Salesman* and *The Cherry Orchard*, for example, plays that I will examine later, present the kind of information about family interaction that might take a good therapist a number of sessions to unpack.

Plays offer us then the opportunity to examine and analyse. They can also trigger powerful emotional reactions. Ever since the first censorship debate – between Aristotle and Plato – the power of drama to disturb and influence us in its capacity to reflect our lives (mimesis) has remained an undisputed truth. Whether or not that influence was healthy was the subject of the two philosophers' disagreement. Plato's concern was that drama had a terrible power to corrupt; he disapproved of the excesses of emotion and lack of manly restraint that drama could evoke. His stern view was that theatre encouraged emotional indulgence and with it, moral weakness. Conversely, Aristotle extolled the purifying power of drama, specifically tragedy, through its emotional and spiritual release or catharsis. He believed this catharsis was produced through the spectator's identification with the action and characters and this in turn evoked the dual emotions of pity and fear (empathy). The spectators feel pity for the protagonist's misfortune and recognize fear that this too could be their fate. However, as this takes place on the stage, the spectators can go through the experience vicariously. Using Aristotle's idea, theatre becomes a site for the audiences' 'projections'.

This immediate emotional experience that theatre affords us is an important one. As therapists we are rightly expected to contain the emotional responses that client families might arouse in us and then of course to analyse and understand them. Our emotional world is processed through cognitive filters. If an elderly family member sat with me in an interview and declared that he belonged to the past and that it was time for his children to move on towards the future and for him to die, I would not cry. I would perhaps think of my own grandfather: remember doing up the top button of his shirt for him because his fingers were to weak; remember filling in his pools form for him; remember how my family fell apart when he died. But I would not cry in the session. I might instead discuss this personal aspect afterwards with a consultant or supervisor. When, at the end of *The Cherry Orchard*, Firs, the loyal old family retainer who has been left behind and forgotten, mutters to himself: 'You silly old nothing' and rocks and falls off his chair, presumably to die, then I cry. And in so doing I demonstrate with some immediacy my own emotional connections with Chekhov's script about change and loss.

A play offers us then the opportunity to watch the experiences of others from a distance and we can both empathize and analyse. We can examine what is going on and consider the scripts that are being played out and we can experience and identify our own emotional reactions. And because the action is 'over there' on stage or screen with no organizing context of responsibility, no requirement for us to be helpful, and because the feelings are once removed, then they are less threatening and we are more able to consider them with an openness and interest.

The colloquial dramas of television series such as *EastEnders* can provide helpful triggers. A friend of mine lost his mother. He couldn't find ways of sharing his grief with his partner and instead became difficult and retreated from the relationship. His partner was too distressed by what was happening to the relationship to be able to connect with his friend's emotional state. They were at risk of separating. All this, until they both watched an episode of *EastEnders* where an elderly female character died. My bereaved friend wept and was comforted by his partner. A new conversation and a healing process began. On another occasion a woman I had been seeing for some time following her husband's suicide, arrived in my office distressed because her teenage daughter had become pregnant and had had an abortion. We explored what this meant to the family and my client reiterated the view that she felt a failure and abnormal ever since her husband's death; that all her friends had normal family lives with husbands and well-behaved children and it was only hers that was strange. We discussed the concept of normality and I asked her if she had seen the film *American Beauty*, a film that deals in part with a caricature of suburban normality and all that this disguises. She smiled and understood. This moved us on so we could use the scripts of the families in *American Beauty* as a way of highlighting the differences in my client's family script – for example, the very open and communicative relationship she has with her daughter. In sharing an understanding of *American Beauty* we were able to use the film as a shared metaphor.

Drama: 'the depiction of reality for the purpose of influencing reality'

You artists who, for pleasure or for pain
Deliver yourselves up to the judgement of the audience
Be moved in future
To deliver up also to the judgement of the audience
The world which you show.

Brecht (1976)

Dramatists like therapists have their strategies and interventions to help bring about change by encouraging audiences to explore their world from different perspectives. In this respect the contribution of the great German writer and director Bertolt Brecht is significant. Brecht energetically propounded an alternative view to Aristotle's emotional, dramatic theatre. He believed that drama should provoke our thinking and some of his theories foreshadow the ideas of systemic therapists, notably the Milan team.

Brecht thought that theatre should help people to change their lives and their society and, therefore, should be instructive. His view was that so long as audiences were identifying with the emotional component of the drama they were, in effect, spellbound and unable to be critically detached and evaluative. He urged that theatre should develop ways of 'alienating' the audience so that they were not caught up in an emotional identification with the characters on stage, and thus entranced by that emotion. Brecht coined the term *Verfremdungseffekt* to describe these devices for creating alienation. Through the use of this *Verfremdungseffekt*, the audience was invited to notice things in a new way, to be jolted into seeing as strange, situations and conditions from a socio-political perspective that they had previously taken for granted.

Systemic therapists will recognize the same concern to create a helpful *Verfremdungseffekt* by working with a team and having team members observe and consult to the therapy 'as audience' from another room. Equally circular questioning reveals and perturbs the *status quo* of a family belief system and so invites family members to consider each other in new ways.

Brecht's theatre was deeply political in its concern with change. Because his project was to show how historical and social contexts determined the scripts by which people were encouraged to live, he created an Epic form for his theatre:

> Today [1931] when human character must be understood as the 'totality of all social conditions' the epic form is the only one that can comprehend all the processes, which could serve the drama as materials for a fully representative picture of the world. (Brecht, quoted in Esslin, 1984)

Because Brecht's theatre was rooted in a political context, it was interested in the way social context determined the interactions between people. Characters were vehicles for the story (or *fabel*), that being:

> 'The sequence of events which constitutes the social experiment of the play; it provides the dialectical field for the interplay of social forces from which the lesson of the play will be seen to emerge' (Esslin, 1984).

And each scene of the play was built around a particular *gestus*: what Martin Esslin refers to as 'the whole range of the outward signs of social relationships ... the clear and stylised expression of the social behaviour of human beings towards each other' (ibid.).

Brecht had his actors perform in such a way that they somehow *narrated* their characters rather than inhabited them. This meant that in terms of their script they had to convey to the audience that this was not the only script available to their character. There were alternatives: their characters had made a choice and could equally make a different one. This acting style sought to expose the distinctions between the actors, their character, and their characters' actions and so to make conscious the playmaking process and the relationship between actors and audience. In John Byng-Hall's terms, Brecht's aim was to offer to audiences a vision of 'corrective' scripts.

Brecht's privileging of thinking over feeling in the quest for change was certainly the position the influential Milan school took when I first started training. Then we were discouraged from asking clients how they felt. We were more interested in eliciting 'The clear and stylised expression of the social behaviour of human beings towards each other' (op. cit.) via circular questioning. We were not encouraged to enter personal therapy to explore our own responses and feelings. Instead a team was located behind the screen to help us 'manage' our feelings so that we could think more constructively. Reflexivity is now at the heart of more recent developments in this area. It has helped to bring feelings and the personal world of the therapist back into the frame and helped us to look at the ways that we are often likely to be provoked intellectually by something that first connects with us emotionally.

Dario Fo, the political Italian dramatist, was very aware of the reflexive relationship between stage and audience and used this to make audiences think. He saw the theatre 'as a great machine which makes people laugh at dramatic things ... In the laughter there remains a sediment of anger' (quoted by Hanna in Rame and Fo, 1990). When I performed in a play by him and his then partner, Franca Rame, about gender relations, my task was to push the comedy until the audience was on my side, crying with laughter. Then suddenly I had to change tack; to separate myself from that laughter and to undercut it with a grim line of 'truth'. This was designed to destabilize the audience and make them look at themselves and question the whole premise upon which their laughter was based.

Imagination

I am aware that the discussion so far has focussed on the play as a performance. Text analysis can like an analysis of a case transcript make for dry reading. Analysis leaches the life out of a play: the passions of the characters, the atmosphere and moods of each scene disappear under the micro-scope. It is the reader's imagination that can bring all this back to life. The imaginative process is a vital part of any discussion about the shared metaphor of theatre. It is embedded in the reflexive relationship of client and therapist as surely as it is embedded in the relationship between playwright, actor and audience.

While in our training and literature we attend rigorously to the empirical aspect of our task, the role of imagination remains largely unexplored. In privileging the science of our work we neglect that creative faculty. This is curious: perhaps we think it unimportant, or maybe we do not yet have the language to discuss it. Our imagination contributes much to our under-standing of clients' stories. How else do we 'see' what they mean when they describe their situation and relationships if not via our imagination – our 'mind's eye'? We use the term 'narrative therapy' and talk about clients' stories but rarely examine in those conversations the crucial part the imagi-nation has always played in telling stories and listening to stories. When we meet clients shouldn't we instinctively start creating set designs in our heads as they talk? See their home; their parent's home; their work environment; visualize the characters and the scenes? Each question we ask helps to develop the moving pictures, the play that we construct in our imagination.

Scripts

The notion of scripts is at the core of John Byng-Hall's use of the theatre metaphor. We think of a script as something that tells an actor how their character speaks and behaves; what their character says. The word in itself refers to writing: a text, something more or less fixed which the actor learns. So every time she or he plays a specific part or role, their script is the same.

This idea of a script as something fixed and something learned is an important aspect of the metaphor. John Byng-Hall defines family scripts as 'the family's shared expectations of how family roles are to be performed within various contexts' (Byng-Hall, 1995b). He uses the term to describe how ways of being and relating are learned in families over generations and can become fixed and repetitive. 'If they complain about how the same situation arises again and again, we are soon likely to find ourselves talking about scripts' and he coins the term 'family scenario' to describe this repeating situation. Such a family scenario comprises a context in which the family interaction occurs, a plot – meaning 'the way family members "motives" become clear as the scenario unfolds' – and an outcome, the consequences of the interaction. Byng-Hall points out that usually family members anticipate early on in the scenario where it is going to end. They know their roles in the piece and they have witnessed and been party to the same kind of situation many times before. Often their attempts to influence or change the direction of the scenario can lead to a situation whereby the attempted solution becomes the problem.

In the following discussions of Arthur Miller's *Death of a Salesman* (1949) and Anton Chekhov's play *The Cherry Orchard* (Chekhov, 1904), I want to look at the way some of these aspects of family scripts are exposed – how, for example, each playwright has used specific tools to present these areas and to make them serve the story. This is after all an important point of departure for therapist and playwright. Therapists collect information in order to construct a story with their clients. Playwrights know the story and must present the information in all its complexity in ways that meaningfully share that story with their audience.

The first area to examine is context, how each play has been situated and structured in order to expose intended meanings. This includes the way family myths are used to bring family history into the frame. The second area is the interaction, the scripts themselves. Here I want to look at the way change functions in each play and how 'replicative' and 'corrective' scripts trace that trajectory of change towards an outcome.

Context

> Context is the key tool of the dramatist. Relationships between one scene and the next, between one line and the next, between what is being said and what is being done are among the chief weapons in the writer's armoury. A man tells you he never eats whilst making himself a sandwich, cries whilst saying he is happy, laughs after being shot. (Anthony Minghella)

In his paper, 'The Family in Modern Drama', Arthur Miller is clear that all great plays address the following key questions:

> How may a man make of the outside world a home? How and in what way must he struggle? What must he strive to change and overcome within himself and outside himself if he is to find the safety, the surroundings of love, the ease of soul, the sense of identity and honour which evidently all men have connected in their memories with the idea of family? (Miller, 1956)

Here then is another place where dramatists and systemic therapists meet; a concern to look at the relationship between human beings and their environment, defined and given meaning by their understanding of family. Both Anton Chekhov and Arthur Miller addressed these questions in their work. In *The Cherry Orchard* Chekhov looked at the impact of a changing society on a family. In *Death of a Salesman* Miller used one man's sense of family to explore his struggle to meet what he perceives to be the demands of the American

Dream. So how did these playwrights bring context on to the stage and show us the relationship between individual, family and the 'outside world'?

Culture, class and history are significant overarching contexts in both plays. Chekhov was a reformer. He wanted to help people see the changes that were happening in his country in the nineteenth century. He wanted to help them meet those changes, and he did it by showing them what the experience of going through change looked like. Drama students tell me they dislike Chekhov because 'he's so boring, nothing happens in his plays'. Indeed nothing very dramatic does happen and essentially that is because in many of his plays, *The Cherry Orchard* is a prime example, people are doing little but waiting – recognizing what Trevor Griffiths calls the 'objective necessity' (Chekhov, 1978) of change and waiting for it to take its course. Equally Chekhov understood that change could occur at the most inconsequential moment and with the minimum of fuss. His project as a playwright was to commit this to the stage:

> Let everything on the stage be just as complicated, and at the same time just as simple as it is in life. People eat their dinner, just eat their dinner ... and at the same time their happiness is being established or their lives are being broken.
> (Chekhov, quoted by Hingley, 1966)

In realising this, Chekhov used symbolic references to great effect. In *The Cherry Orchard* he describes the context of a changing society, positioning particular characters carefully in the play. The structure of the play's beginning and end vividly demonstrates this. It starts with Lophakin, the voice of a new emerging bourgeois society, shaking himself awake to greet Mme Ranevskaya and her family as they arrive by train. The play ends with Firs the ancient family retainer, the symbolic character from the 'old regime', left behind and falling asleep, to die, as the family departs following the sale of the estate. 'The future' wakes up and introduces the play, and with the end of the play, the past dies (Alan Pearlman, 1992).

The Cherry Orchard: case history

Family history

Mme Ranevskaya married a lawyer, a man who gambled and drank and who was not seen as her social equal. As a result, Ranevskaya was disinherited by her aunt. There were two children of the marriage, Grisha and Anya. Ranevskaya's husband died of drink and she embarked on an affair with a man she claimed was 'his double'. While she was engaged in this affair her son Grisha was drowned in a river on the family estate.

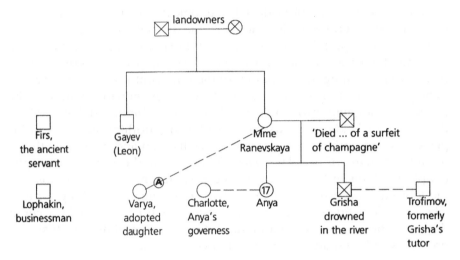

Figure 6.1 Mme Ranevskaya's family and community (*The Cherry Orchard*).

Ranevskaya ran away to France leaving behind her daughter and lover. Her lover followed her and when he fell ill Ranevskaya nursed him for three years, only then to be robbed and abandoned by him. Anya came to Paris accompanied by her governess, Charlotte. Ranevskaya, desperately homesick for Russia, returns with them to the estate. Ranevskaya's brother Gayev has joined them.

Significant others

The estate has been looked after in the meantime by three servants and by Varya, Ranevskaya's adopted daughter. Varya is in love with Lophakin, a local businessman, who grew up on the estate where his father had been a serf. Peter Trofimov has recently arrived. He was Grisha's tutor. He is an eternal student and he and Anya are in love.

Presenting problem

The family estate is about to be sold to pay off debts. Ranevskaya and Gayev have no practical solutions about what they can do to save the estate, although they are desperate not to lose it. Lophakin wants Ranevskaya to have the cherry orchard cut down and the land developed for holiday cottages. Ranevskaya and Gayev are utterly against this but seem to be incapable of mobilizing any resources of their own, though the auction date for the sale is imminent.

Hypotheses

1. In conjunction with the whole country, the family is going through a transition and the prospect of considerable loss. The resources they would normally draw on, such as money, servants good manners and charm, are absent or serve only to help them wait.
2. Ranevskaya is in a state of grief over all the losses in her life. These losses are paralysing the whole system.

Family mythology

Family mythology describes how families understand themselves. This mythology develops over time and within a social and cultural context and provides 'a blueprint for action' (Byng-Hall, 1995b) . This action is what John Byng-Hall calls 'the family script'.

A therapist learns about a family's sense of themselves by exploring the stories family members tell about previous generations and looking at how family beliefs have developed. In this way, a therapist may learn with the family how family mythology contributes to current situations becoming stuck and problematic. Playwrights demonstrate the motivation behind the scripts of particular characters for exactly the same reason. They want to show how the past has helped to shape belief systems that are influencing their characters' scripts and contributing to the drama that is the play.

In *The Cherry Orchard* the family has a powerful sense of its mythology. Chekhov uses Ranevskaya's and Gayev's relationship with the house and orchard to demonstrate this. The family's beloved cherry orchard represents the past: family, childhood, innocence – a sense of order and place. Along with the estate the orchard is to be sold and may be cut down. As the characters wait, we watch them interact, playing out their different scripts, arguing their beliefs and different positions in the context of a changing Russia and a dying class. Ranevskaya and Gayev are deeply sentimental and hark back to the past: she with tender melancholy and he with fatuous rhetoric.

As the family reunite in their old family home. Gayev places his hands on the sides of the bookcase and remarks that it is a hundred years old; that they should celebrate its centenary. He then delivers an absurd speech that caricatures his family and the mythology that has shaped it:

> My dear, honoured bookcase. I salute your life. For one hundred years you have borne witness to the noble ideals of goodness and of justice. For one hundred

years your silent call to hard work has sounded in the ears of generation upon generation of this our family, sustaining us in our moments of weakness, strengthening in us our belief in a better tomorrow, and implanting in us the moral idea of virtue and the moral idea of social order.

In his discussion of how family myths function John Byng-Hall points out that: 'One danger is that a family myth may become a closed belief system, unable to integrate new information. This is particularly likely to happen if the family feels that a challenge to its beliefs threatens its very survival' (Byng-Hall, 1995). Here is a problem that goes straight to the heart of the play. Family survival is already an issue for Ranevskaya and Gayev so, although new information is available, they cannot accommodate it. It is too threatening.

As therapists we learn to explore difference, to look, for example, for the alternative views within or outside the family, that may have some influence on a problem, either in bringing about change or in impeding change. It is also important for a therapist to understand why a family cannot 'see' alternatives that may be helpful or feel that they cannot access the alternatives. A dramatist has similarly to identify the alternative positions, because it is often in the light of these that conflict or the family drama is exposed.

In *The Cherry Orchard*, Lophakin, serf turned businessman, represents the future, the 'new order'. Ranevskaya and Gayev reject his suggestions for modernizing their estate through commercial enterprise. They would rather lose their land than submit to change. Bearing in mind Cronen and Pearce's hierarchy of contexts (1985), which proposes a layering of defining contexts, the 'act of communication' which captures this essence of the play can clearly be seen in the following dialogue between Mme Ranevskaya, Gayev and Lophakin:

L: I'm trying not to give offence but you two must be just about the most reckless and feckless people I have ever met. You're told in words of one syllable – you are about to lose your land – and it seems to make no impression.

R: But what can we do about it? Have you an answer?

L: I give you the answer every single day, there is only one answer; the orchard and the land down to the river must be leased out for summer cottages And it must be done now, the auction's almost upon us. Do you understand?

He looks from one to the other. Mme R has removed a shoe to stroke the arch of her foot. Gayev chalks his cue with languid precision

R: Summer cottages, weekenders – it's all so 'bourgeois'.

Yet as Lophakin goes to march off she calls him back beseechingly:

R: Please. I beg of you. It's always so much cheerier when you're with us.

The stage directions for the actors combined with the script succinctly demonstrate the family myth at work when faced with the bourgeois solution. Because of their class and upbringing, Ranevskaya and her brother Gayev are incapable of taking decisions or action. The assumption bred into them is that 'someone will provide'. A vivid feature of their script is: 'We are charming, loving and entertaining, but not functional.' Time and again Lophakin entreats the family to meet change and to deal with it and time and again they reject this possibility. It is Ranevskaya's daughter, Anya, who changes the family script.

Replicative and corrective scripts

Replicative and corrective scripts are different types of transgenerational family scripts (Byng-Hall, 1995b). Essentially they refer to how the experience of family is taken by children and recreated in the next generation. Although John Byng-Hall discusses these scripts in his book largely in terms of how children repeat or change parenting scripts, he is referring to a more general position about allegiance to or differentiation from the family script. Thus a corrective script signifies the rule: 'I must be different' (personal communication). As shown, characters can be positioned to symbolize or highlight an aspect of the play, and the children in *The Cherry Orchard* (and *Death of a Salesman*) have an important function in this respect. Their declarations of difference from their families signify the change that has happened in the course of each play. Consistent with the tone of the play Anya gently assumes her new beliefs and values without struggle or interference from her mother or uncle. Out of the sad acceptance of the death of the old order, she emerges as a new voice, the voice of the future and the way ahead.

We learn from the start of the play that Anya is very different from her mother and uncle. Her tone with them is parental. In her description of her mother's situation we gain some sense of the childlike incapacity that is the birthright of this family – a family born to servants and unlimited wealth:

> We arrive in Paris ... mother's living in a fifth floor apartment and when I arrive she has some French people, some ladies, an old priest with a bible in his hand, the room's dingy and full of smoke. I just suddenly – I felt so sorry for her – I just suddenly took mama's head in my hands and held on tight and couldn't let go. And mama ... hugged me. Cried.

Anya comforts her mother on more than one occasion like a parent comforting a child and she tells her uncle off for talking too much and being disloyal. This parentified behaviour serves to reinforce the childlike qualities of Ranevskaya and Gayev but also suggests that with Anya's more capable and responsible attitude the family script of charming helplessness is changing. This is further reinforced when Anya becomes attached to Trofimov, the 'progressive' intellectual who embraces the future and rejects utterly all that Ranevskaya and Gayev represent. Trofimov introduces Anya to a new set of beliefs and a new understanding about the past. To him the cherry orchard represents the slavery and exploitation of the serfs by the landowners. In one of his edifying speeches to Anya he describes this:

> Our orchard is all of Russia ... Mmm? This vast amazing continent, think of all the fine places there are in it. And think of something else Anya; Your father's father, and his father, and his, were owners of serfs. They owned human lives, Anya. From every tree in your orchard, there are people hanging, they peer at you through the branches, you can hear their voices moaning in the leaves. Owning other human beings is what has destroyed your line – those who came before, those who live on – so that your mother, your uncle you yourself still can't quite grasp that you're living and always have lived off the sweat and labour of someone else.

Here then is the voice, arguably Chekhov's own, foreshadowing the revolution that was to change Russia's history. Notice how significantly it compares to Gayev's speech to the bookcase – a very different rendering on the same theme of the past.

Death of a Salesman

Death of a Salesman, written almost fifty years later and on another continent, deals with a similar theme to that of *The Cherry Orchard* – a family that is out of place, out of kilter with the times. In both cases survival is an issue, survival of the family and the family belief system in changing times. Arthur Miller's declared project in writing the play was to show life through context:

> I aimed to make a play with the veritable countenance of life. To make one the many, as in life, so that 'society' is a power and a mystery of custom and inside the man and surrounding him, as the fish is in the sea and the sea inside the fish. (1988)

Look in the very first instance at the way Miller describes his set:

Before us is the salesman's house. We are aware of towering angular shapes behind it, surrounding it on all sides. Only the blue light of the sky falls upon the house; the surrounding area shows an angry glow of

*orange. As more light appears we see a solid vault of apartment houses
around the small fragile-seeming home. An air of the dream clings to the
place, a dream rising out of reality.*

As Miller locates the Loman family physically so he gives that location a
meaning through the juxtaposing of buildings and the use of different
lighting. He begins to reveal a context of alienation. He shows the old
being overpowered by the new. He brings to mind the small and fragile
being overpowered by all that is progressive and aggressive. Here too
there is a resonance of small town, cap-in-hand subservience, juxtaposed
against tough and modern pushiness. In his play Miller sets the cultural
mythology of the American Dream against the Loman family's belief
system and in this set description, the first contextual marker of the play,
that relationship is given some definition.

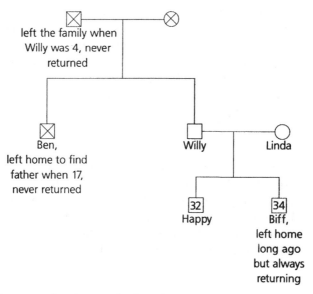

Figure 6.2 The Loman family (*Death of a Salesman*).

Family history

Willy Loman is a salesman. His family is second generation American Jewish
immigrants. He is married to Linda and they have two sons, Biff and Happy.
Willy had an older brother Ben who is now dead. When Willy was four his
father left home. When Ben was seventeen he set off to find their father in
Alaska and ended up in Africa. Willy was brought up on his own, by his
mother. Biff has left home a number of times, always after rows with his

father, but always returns. Willy wants his boys to be a success and is frightened that Biff is a failure. Linda is very protective and supportive of Willy.

Significant others

Charley is Willy's friend and neighbour. A successful man, he lends Willy money and has offered him a job which Willy has refused. Charley's son Bernard grew up with Biff and Happy and allowed them to copy his work and cheat off him at school. He also worried when they stole and did things that might get them in trouble. Bernard is now a successful lawyer.

Presenting problem

Willy Loman is not making any sales and feels a failure. He is not bringing any money in to the family. He is on the verge of a breakdown, and thinking about suicide so that his wife can redeem his insurance policy. He keeps remembering the past and seeing his brother talking to him. His son Biff has returned home and Willy sees his sons' failures as a mirror of his own. Willy carries a guilty secret. In his attempts to be successful in his job, he had an affair with the secretary of one of his larger customers that was largely responsible for securing him sales. His guilt over the affair haunts him and is compounded by the fact that his son Biff, who had idolized him as a child, discovered the affair.

Hypotheses

For Willy Loman the attempted solution has become the problem. The more he has tried to achieve success, according to his perception of the American Dream, the greater his failure. The 'salesman' belief system colours and shapes every aspect of his life and self. Willy's sons seem to be following the same pattern. Biff has a leaving home problem. He cannot get on with his life until he is reconciled with his father and the issue of his father's affair.

In *Death of a Salesman*, the American Dream of mid-twentieth century America is the significant cultural context. 'A man who works hard can have everything the country has to offer; can be the king of his own empire.' But working hard isn't enough to bring success to a travelling salesman; Willy Loman has worked hard but the dream has eluded him.

Here with the Lomans we see the very antithesis of Ranevskaya's family belief in *The Cherry Orchard*. The Loman family script is about an immigrant group struggling to find a way of belonging and to leave a mark; trying to work out the rules for success as they go along and finding that they keep going wrong. As Willy says in despair to his wife Linda:

> 'I don't know why – I can't stop myself – I talk too much. A man oughta come in
> with a few words. One thing about Charley. He's a man of few words and they
> respect him ... I joke too much ...'

Willy's final gesture to provide for his family is entirely consistent with his
understanding of a salesman's rules: you are your own asset. Finally, tragically, with his suicide he achieves success. He sells himself for the price of
his life insurance.

Family myths

Death of a Salesman is a play built around the mythology that helped to
create America. The Loman family myths are fed by that context. The Loman
men are continually asserting these myths in terms of their rules and injunctions about what it means to be a man and how a man ought to live. For
Willy, whose father disappeared when he was very young, these rules a have
been beacons to see him through his life. They are now props to support
him as he feels himself coming apart. For his son Biff they are statements of
dissatisfaction and arguments for change. When Biff angrily declares:

> They've laughed at dad for years, and you know why? Because we don't belong
> in this nuthouse of a city! We should be mixing cement on some open plain, or
> – or carpenters. A carpenter is allowed to whistle!

he is giving voice to a Loman family myth based on the family's immigrant
history about the great outdoors – where they really belong.

Miller emphasizes the family myths in this play by bringing the past on
stage in the form of Willy Loman's dead brother, Ben, the person who in
Willy's mind represents the success of the family myths. Stories are told
about Ben. We don't know what is true. It is only through the eyes of
Willy's wife Linda that the unpleasant, exploitative sides of Ben and this
myth of the American Dream are exposed.

As with the family in *The Cherry Orchard*, the Lomans have a potential
solution to their predicament. Willy's kindly friend and neighbour Charley
has been bailing Willy out for a long time, lending him money. He is the
possibility of a father figure, the mentor that Willy never had. And
although Willy will borrow money from Charley he refuses the job offer
that would secure his future. In this stubborn refusal to accept proper
help, Willy is asserting a rule born of the family myth that 'men have to
make it on their own'. Similarly, the uncritical love and support that Willy's
wife Linda offers her husband counts for naught with him. In its attention
to social and cultural contexts *Death of a Salesman* deals with relationships between men in a climate defined by male values. Crucially,

however, it is Linda's interventions throughout the play that finally effect the reconciliation between father and son.

Replicative and corrective scripts

In *Death of a Salesman* the themes of struggle and misunderstanding colour the whole matter of the inheritance of the family script. This focuses on Biff, the older son. Biff has 'run away' from home, so replicating the family script. Willy's father ran away from home and Willy's brother left home to seek his fortune; both were mythologized and idealized. Unlike his grandfather and uncle, though, Biff keeps coming back to his family, only to squabble with his father and leave again.

Having set up a problematic relationship between Willy and Biff, Miller then repeatedly shows the family script in action. We see the Loman males trying desperately to show each other that they are achieving and then being reduced by the pathos of their lies, deceits and failures. Miller cranks up the tension by bringing Biff home at the point when Willy is breaking down and contemplating suicide. This time Biff can't solve the problem with his father by leaving. Something has to change. It isn't until towards the end of the play, when Biff confronts his father about Willy's preparations for suicide that he names the game and exposes the script as hollow:

Biff   (*to Happy, about Willy*): The man doesn't know who we are! The
        man is gonna know! (To Willy) We never told the truth for ten
        minutes in this house!

Then he starts to tell the truth:

Biff: I stole myself out of every good job since High School.
Willy: And whose fault is that?
Biff: And I never got anywhere because you blew me so full of hot air I
        could never stand taking orders from anybody. That's whose fault it
        is!

Later he pleads with his father to let go of the American Dream:

Biff: I am not a leader of men, Willy, and neither are you. You were
        never anything but a hard working drummer who landed in the ash
        can, like all the rest of them. I'm one dollar an hour, Willy. I tried
        seven states and couldn't raise it. A buck an hour. Do you gather
        my meaning? I'm not bringing home any prizes any more and
        you're going to stop waiting for me to bring them home!

Then 'at the peak of his fury' he breaks down:

Biff: Pop. I'm nothing. I'm nothing pop. Can't you understand that? There's no spite in it any more. I'm just what I am that's all.

His father is astonished at his son's crying. Here is the new information that makes the difference. In this honest declaration and through his tears, Biff is connecting more powerfully with his father than he ever has.

Linda: He loves you Willy.
Willy: Oh Biff. *Staring wildly* He cried! Cried to me.

Willy's realisation that his son loves him is an extraordinarily poignant moment in the play. It is an act of communication that cuts through all the rules the men have learned about 'what it means to be a man'. It is a change in the family script that is forced into being.

Conclusion

> There is a powerful case for an art form which can never dissolve the scale of the human figure, the sound of the human voice and our desire to tell each other stories.
>
> (Richard Eyre, 2001)

In this chapter I have sought to extend the 'shared metaphor' and to look at the conjunctions between theatre and therapy from different perspectives, with a view to exploring the potential for more creative and imaginative therapy. What I have found is that some striking features emerge, as much from the differences as from the similarities between the two worlds. Each investigates the tragedies and comedies of our lives, but one uses the public domain and the other the private. The public space of theatre is a safer space for it does not engage us immediately in pressures of personal responsibility. It is after all a place of entertainment. The theatre tells us stories and at the same time it can challenge us both emotionally and intellectually. This is evident in the plays I have analysed.

The theatre is a place of possibility and enchantment. It offers therapists a system of values that can function as an antidote to the potentially oppressive nature of therapy and can provide tools and a new vocabulary. Whilst plays may be thought provoking and deeply moving, the world of the theatre encourages us to play and to be imaginative; with play and creativity come new perspectives.

It seems to me that a key to the shared metaphor is the theatre's capacity to help us to look at ourselves – however, we choose. Theatre is a mirror that we hold up to ourselves so that we become simultaneously observer and observed. In that reflexive relationship there is a great deal to be explored.

Kate Daniels works as a systemic psychotherapist in a general practice and teaches on the Postgraduate Diploma in Applied Systemic Theory at the Tavistock Clinic. She studied drama and comparative literature at the University of Kent, where she taught playwriting, and she did postgraduate work with playwright David Edgar at Birmingham University. Her roles as an actor include Beatrice in Much Ado About Nothing, *Emma in Harold Pinter's* Betrayal *and Lady Fidget in the restoration comedy* A Country Wife. *Her last job before leaving acting to concentrate on writing was with a national tour of* A Little Like Drowning, *a semi-autobiographical play by Anthony Minghella.*

Chapter 7
Death, family scripts and systemic existentialism

John Hills

His father gave him a box of truisms
Shaped like a coffin, then his father died;
The truisms remained on the mantelpiece
As wooden as the playbox they had been packed in
Or that other his father skulked inside.

Then he left home, left the truisms behind him
Still on the mantelpiece, met love, met war,
Sordor, disappointment, defeat, betrayal,
Till through disbeliefs he arrived at a house
He could not remember seeing before,

And he walked straight in; it was where he had come from
And something told him the way to behave.
He raised his hand and blessed his home;
The truisms flew and perched on his shoulders
And a tall tree sprouted from his father's grave.

>   (Louis Macneice, 'The Truisms' *Selected Poems*, 1988)

What is the self? ... The self is a relation which relates itself to its own self. Man is a synthesis of the infinite and the finite, of the temporal and the eternal, of freedom and necessity, in short, it is a synthesis. (Kierkegaard, 1843)

When an experience is, or has been intolerable, the family may defend itself by avoiding the situations in which either the affect or the action may arise. This may be called the family defence ... Every family needs some defence. (Byng-Hall, 1982b)

Introduction

Systemic psychotherapy is, as described in the Preface, a generic approach to psychotherapy based on systemic thinking. It is both a process analysis and synthesis of lived experience, and a conceptual psychotherapeutic schema which incorporates some of the diverse conceptual hypotheses about problem formation and change in other therapies, re-presenting them from a different perspective in a completely new framework. At the centre of this schema is the interest in understanding patterns of organization of the intersubjective, and the active pursuit of the meaning of change of such patterns.

In brief, for it has a large and growing literature, it uses at least six *domains of human experience,* three *keystone principles of thinking* and three basic *modes of intervention.* The six domains of experience, whether overt or submerged and which guide and inform the therapist's use of the three modes of intervention (*directing, interactive questioning* and *open reflecting*) in the therapeutic dialogue are *emotion and feeling; transaction and communication; belief and thinking; the problem/solution paradoxes and their strategies; narrative and the construction of meaning; boundary, structure and alliance* (e.g. Fleuridas et al., 1986; Tomm, 1988; Corey and Bitter, 1996; Brown, 1997). Though these are described as if discrete domains, in practice they intertwine and direct the therapist's thinking and focus. Systemic psychotherapy has few insights that are not shared with other therapies, but the totality of the approach is quite distinctive and different.

Only the three keystone principles of thinking that give systemic psychotherapy this distinctiveness will be the discussed here. These are: *its understanding of the holonistic nature of reality; the enantriodromic or homeostatic tendency in all systems and in experienced reality;* and *the systemic context.* Taken together these give a very different perspective on family processes and on the 'process' of being a person. All people are located somewhere, in a total environment with a background and a foreground. They move and have their being, with different degrees of awareness, through the outcome of their intentions, their choosing, their feeling and reciprocal interaction with their environment of others. This is the intersubjectivity of human relations. Human beings are organized in and by many systems which serve to define relationships with one another. These systems form part of the total ecosphere and multiversity of the planet. Our individual psychology can also be seen as a personal ecology of being; our existence is both a systemic fact and a systemic experience.

The principle of holonistic thinking

This rather unattractive neologism was first coined by the Hungarian-born philosopher and novelist, Arthur Koestler. It represents a significant contribution to systemic thought, though only the family therapist Salvador Minuchin has used it (Minuchin and Fishman, 1981). The fact that our universe is organized in a concatenation of interconnecting systems was articulated clearly four centuries ago by the French mathematician Blaise Pascal (1670):

> There is, for example, a relationship between man and all he knows ... since all things are both caused and causing, assisted and assisting ... providing mutual support in a chain linking together ... the most distant and different things, I consider it as impossible to know the parts without knowing the whole as to know the whole without knowing the individual parts.

Just as a finger is a 'whole' object in own right, so it is simultaneously a 'part' object – of a hand, arm, shoulder, or body, etc. This is its holonistic property; its 'wholepartness' or 'partwholeness'. It is the basic building block of all systems, from a car assembly line, circulatory system of the human body, educational system, sewage system, to the system of this chapter in this book. Systems may be organized horizontally, like a web, or hierarchically, like a tree. However, Koestler makes clear (1975) that the use of the word 'hierarchy' is used here descriptively, in the same way that systemic psychotherapists understand it when drawing genograms:

> We find such tree diagrams of hierarchic organization applied to the most varied fields: genealogical tables; the classification of animals and plants; the evolutionist's 'tree of life'; charts indicating the branching structures of government departments or industrial enterprizes; physiological charts of the nervous system and of the circulation of the blood. The word 'hierarchy' is of ecclesiastical origin and is often wrongly used to refer merely to order of rank ...

When holonistic thinking is applied to the idea of 'the person' or 'individuality', it gives a different perspective to other psychotherapy theories of intersubjectivity, such as 'object relations'. While holonistic thinking in no way detracts from the uniqueness of the person, it prefers to locate this uniqueness in the systems of relationships which nurture, protect and develop identity and of which the human family is the most proximate and intimate. Koestler maintains the wholeness of the person ('the individual') is simultaneously embedded in the partness of others ('the dividual'). Family relationships in their systemic form are thus embedded in each other. He likens this simultaneity to the ancient god Janus whose statue the Romans often placed in entrances: two-headed, Janus faced both inside the home and outside. He symbolically represents the tension of holonistic thinking, inclusive or exclusive, according to how it is perceived. Koestler (1980) expressed this simultaneous 'partwholeness',' wholepartness' thus:

> No man is an island; he is a holon. Looking inward, he experiences himself as a unique, self-contained, independent whole; looking outward as a dependent part of his natural and social environment. His self-assertive tendency is the dynamic manifestation of his individuality; his integrative tendency expresses his dependence on some larger whole to which he belongs, his partness. When all is well, the two tendencies are more or less evenly balanced. In times of stress and frustration, the equilibrium is upset, manifested in emotional disorders.

The late Robin Skynner sought to explore this idea in his major family-therapy text *One Flesh Separate Persons* (Skynner, 1976). The term 'the community of internalised others' (widely attributed to Karl Tomm) describes 'the dividual' part of our holonistic being, which informs part of our identity and sense of self. We are in the family and the family is in us. As Teddy put it to his menacing family in Harold Pinter's *The Homecoming* (Pinter, 1978):

> You're just objects. You just ... move about. I can observe it. I can see what you do. It's just the same as I do. But you're lost in it. You won't get me being ... I won't be lost in it.

Each of us is *observer* and *enactor* simultaneously in our intersubjectivity. It is this holonistic tension between these modes of being that underlies the systemic psychotherapist's skill through interactive interviewing.

The enantriodromic principle

Taken from the ancient Greek thinker Heraclitus (*c.* 500 BC), *enantrio-dromia* is the dynamic tension between opposites, often concealed by the appearance of stability. His pre-scientific belief was of a universe in a constant state of flux yet appearing unchanging: 'you can never step into the same river twice'. It is this principle that Koestler describes above in the tension between self-assertiveness and integration. All systems are in part organized to maintain a steady state, or homeostasis, between differences which threaten change. This applies to the stability of a ship, global or body temperature, parties in a political system or different ethnic groups in a community. The Hegelian dialectic of the conflict of ideas between the 'thesis', the 'antithesis' and the emerging 'synthesis' is the philosophical equivalent of the enantriodromic principle. Cybernetics, the control systems in mechanical and biological systems, are based on enantriodromic principles.

Our experienced world, with its awareness of personal characteristics, is also composed of opposites and differences – day and night, male and female, close and distant, passive and aggressive, compliance and defiance, strength and weakness, depression and euphoria, optimism and pessimism, intellect and feeling. Part of the process of individuation is to struggle, both consciously and unconsciously, to find the best location in and reconciliation of such differences. The common notion of psychological ambivalence is the simultaneous coming together of different feelings or contradictory beliefs held together in a difficult tension; denial, disassociation and projection are similarly enantriodromic processes, though always described as if unitary experiences, because that is how they seem. Rigidity of thought and belief usually arise from the anxiety of looking at difference and change and failure to appreciate the workings of enantriodromia. There are also cultural influences on our thinking and beliefs so that ideas of individuation and the development of the person are not always contextually appropriate.

John Byng-Hall's notion of family script is based on the enantriodromic principle – experience is located on a continuum and may be repeated or corrected. Within the intersubjectivity of family relationships, third or fourth members may be involved in regulating the levels of closeness or distance, safety or harm. These patterns are not based solely in the notion of the unconscious but arise from the organization of powerful group emotional tensions. This leads on to the final principle, that of context.

The principle of context

There are various ways 'context' is understood in systemic psychotherapy: as the family life-cycle and its interface with the biological life-cycle; insights from developmental psychology; different levels of social experience based on poverty, social inclusion, ethnicity, class, gender and sexual orientation; and personal differences. This draws on the work of Alfred Adler (Hills, 1999) and also the sociological theories of Pearce and Cronen (1980). Their Co-ordinated Management of Meaning proposes a model in which there are at least six levels of context: socio-cultural beliefs, including local community ones; historical, intergenerational family myths and patterns; life-scripts; current relationships; events and episodes; speech acts. The authors maintain that meaning is governed by two key operations, which restate the holonistic principle (Cronen and Pearce, 1982):

1. hierarchical relationships: two units of meaning are in a hierarchical relationship when one unit forms the context for interpreting the meaning and function of the other;
2. reflexive loops: reflexivity exists whenever two elements in a hierarchy are so organized that each is simultaneously the context for and within the context of the other.

Context, therefore, is the background from which personal and family experience emerge.

One notable and serious omission from the consideration of context is the dimension of life itself. The family, however it may be constructed and conceived, is also the matrix for the core existential developmental theme – the personal progression through life to death. The fact of death absolutely and experientially is the central dilemma of life. We may dismiss certain experiences with a resigned 'That's life, isn't it?', as if the subject were too vast to take in. The energy that comes from the fact of our death is rather like that from the sun – not something we want to stare at for long, as the French aphorist La Rochefoucauld sensibly pointed out (Enright 1983). For the family, it is the most powerful single influence in the creation of the life-script, and of experiential difficulties that may require therapeutic help. Holonistically, the family matrix is reconfigured as its participants die. Death is the absolute given and determined event. Like a bothersome insect, it never quite goes away, and around it the family has always to struggle to find a different reality.

John Byng-Hall supervised my work as a family therapist trainee for two years at the Tavistock Clinic in the early 1980s. Much of what I learned from this experience has remained part of my repertoire as a psychotherapist, not least John's unerring capacity to identify the unspoken issues and gently give them a voice. During my training, he selected a 'trigger' family (McGoldrick, 1982) for me to work with – a two-parent family with two sons, aged 11 and seven, the elder of whom had a speech impediment, a stammer. Though from a different religious and cultural background to my own, they were an almost exact duplicate of my family when I was that age and had a similar dysfluency.

Stammering is a 'symptom' with no agreed origin and which fits many explanatory hypotheses, linear and circular, and yet eludes them all – the genetic, communicational, unconscious, strategic, systemic and structural all have validity. As part of the supervision team experience we had, as usual, looked at my family tree and the incidence of stammering in the family (paternal grandfather, maternal great-uncle and cousin), the stories about them and how they overcame their stammer; how family alliances formed around me, as well as the different meanings of hesitant communication. We also looked at the humour in it, how it organizes other people's responses, for instance in 'helpfully' supplying the word they think you want (usually wrongly!); to the strategy of exaggerating the stammer to avoid oral tests in school (and succeeding in failing French as a result!).

As part of my personal work, I presented a dream I had had under anaesthetic as a four-year-old child. At the time we lived in Karachi, then the capital of Pakistan, on a narrow spit of land called Manora which forms one side of the long sheltered harbour. My father had been seconded to the Pakistan Navy, recently created after independence, to help establish a torpedo factory in the dockyard. While my mother was in hospital elsewhere in the city, about to give birth to my brother, my father took me across the harbour to central Karachi to see a dentist. I needed to have a tooth extracted though at that age, I was not used to my father taking me anywhere.

The Pakistani anaesthetist told me to relax while he would place a white handkerchief over my mouth. Nothing would hurt. As he poured chloroform over the white gauze, I had a dream of ferocious intensity. It was an auditory and visual hallucination in which a hot-air balloon with two people inside the basket ascended into the sky to merge with the sun, which had a face and which seemed to be laughing. There was a powerful throbbing in my head, as if an engine had been engaged and my mouth tasted of a terrible bitter chemical. My father was concerned for me but perturbed at the fuss I was causing the dentist. I had put up quite a performance of screamed defiance and protest. Similar performances were produced at any imagined attempt by my parents to take me into Karachi. From that day onward I spoke with stammer. It took years for the haunting images to subside.

John's perspective on the dream was helpful and his supervision transformed the way I understood my work as a family therapist and myself. This then is the personal root of the reflections in this chapter, and for which La Rochefoucauld's injunction strongly applies!

Death and the existential core of being

Death is the central absolute mystery of human existence. As a biological event it is simple and explicit enough, as the dead parrot owner in the memorable Monty Python sketch protested to the feigned disbelief of the pet-shop owner. Its significance and meaning for an individual is as extensive, complex and unique as the person concerned. A whole branch of

philosophy developed, mostly in the last century, based on an understanding of human subjectivity in the face of the inevitability of death, and
our capacity freely to choose aspects of our being, and take responsibility
for those choices. Called Existentialism, its thinkers (such as the French
philosophers, Jean-Paul Sartre and Gabriel Marcel, the French Algerian
Albert Camus, and the German philosopher, Martin Heidegger) followed
a tradition of thought from the Danish philosopher Soren Kierkegaard,
whose definition of the self begins this chapter. Though largely developed before the Second World War, it was popular in Europe in the
immediate postwar period, for reasons not difficult to discern, given the
mass death, wholesale destruction of communities and unthinkable
social dislocation.

Existentialism has since been somewhat superseded in philosophical
fashion by post-modernism, led by the next generation of again mostly
French philosophers: Jean-François Lyotard, Michel Foucault, Jacques
Derrida and Jean Baudrillard. This, in turn, speaks to the condition of the
post-Cold War world, globalization and mass consumerism and awareness
of cultural relativism (though the essential world problems of war, poverty
and disease have not lessened). It is oversimplistic to assume that with the
ending of the nuclear arms race, death is no longer central to the collective
human consciousness. Even as I re-read this, the terrible events of 11
September in New York have created a different mood about the safety of
our world and our sense of being. However, post-modernism often represents many Existentialist ideas of human subjectivity as if they were its
own, and in rejecting ideas of a 'grand narrative' or 'metanarrative' it has
largely eliminated or subjugated 'death discourse' from its schema. Its
growing application to systemic psychotherapy has inbuilt limitations as a
result, while raising useful challenges about the nature of subjectivity.

Existentialism, according to J. Macquarrie, a leading commentator, can
be defined from its etymology:

> to 'exist' or 'ex-sist' (Latin: *ex-sistere*) meant originally to 'stand out' or
> 'emerge'. Thus the verb probably had a more active feel about it than it has
> now. To exist was to emerge or stand out from the background as something
> really there. Putting it more philosophically, *to exist is to stand out from
> nothing.* (Macquarrie, 1980)

When we think about our existence even for a moment, we are aware of
being between two phases of nothingness (or of 'two long periods of
idleness', the novelist Anthony Burgess once wrote!). This is our existential context: we are indeed an enantiodromic synthesis of the finite and
infinite, of the temporal and eternal, as Kierkegaard's definition puts it.
Non-being or nothingness surrounds human existence and how we fill
that space is in part the basis of our own freedom and choosing. A partner

seeking help for his relationship recently said that the effect of leaving his wife of 19 years and two teenage children to set up home with his childhood friend was 'like falling out of somewhere and into the universe'. His eyes filled with fear and awe as he said this. In a much used expression of Sartre's, existence precedes essence. The central character, a Spanish waiter, in the Ernest Hemingway short story, 'A Clean, Well-Lighted Place', has such a moment of 'emerging' awareness:

> turning off the electric light, he continued the conversation with himself: ... what did he fear? It was not fear or dread. It was a nothing that he knew too well. It was all a nothing and a man was nothing too.

The waiter reworks the Lord's Prayer substituting *nada* (Spanish for nothing) throughout:

> Our nada who art in nada, nada be thy name, thy kingdom nada, thy will be nada in nada as it is in nada. Give us this nada our daily nada, nada us not into nada, but deliver us from nada etc.

It is from 'nada' we are 'thrown into the world', to use an existential figure of speech, and into which we may return at any time, by choice, failure of health, accident or age. Thus death is one of the two greatest human moments, second to birth only in sequence and the greatest challenge to our meaning about ourselves.

As might be expected, exploring the personal and interpersonal meaning of this great anxious mystery is a central concern of psychotherapy. While most theories incorporate ideas about death in their thinking, rarely do they give it a central place, for, with all mystery, it generates impossible questions which admit few answers. Its secret, if secret there be, is not revealed. Psychotherapists are therefore no more privileged or expert than anyone else in understanding death. Like those involved in palliative care, they may understand the process of dying and be highly effective in helping to heal the effects of mourning and loss on the living, but that is the limit of the territory. This has not stopped some psychotherapists from claiming expertise in all the existential mysteries of grief and suffering, rushing in where even angels might prefer caution, and where social beliefs are more 'death denying' and tentative (Rycroft and Perlesz, 2001). Glenda Fredman in her excellent book '*Death Talk*' (Fredman, 1997) points to the double bind the professional helper creates unwittingly for the helped: 'you must talk, but you can't', because of the difficult nature of death.

Though Freud identified *thanatos* (death) and *eros* (love) as the twin central human instincts, his principal interest was with the latter. Death more often appears in theories under the themes of loss, mourning and trauma. Since there are no solutions to death, it is unsurprising that the very vastness, depth and intangibility of the subject subordinates it to 'symptoms, solutions and techniques' talk, for psychotherapy is not a seminar on philosophy. Death is understandably seen as the outcome of failure in most areas of medical and psychotherapeutic intervention. Solution-based therapists can scarcely explore death as a problem solving method and expect to have many patients or to be ethically regarded! Yet, many patients in an acute state of suffering and crisis know that the mystery of death may bring relief and peace, while at the same time recoiling from such a conclusion. However, when acted upon, suicide is almost always experienced as a truly aggressive act of rejection and source of distress to those who remain.

Though Existentialism, with its philosophical concerns about death, made a brief incursion into family systemic psychotherapy (mostly through the work of R.D. Laing), it has been as remarkably absent from this approach as from others, though recent writers have suggested 'the subject of death is the last taboo in the field of family therapy' (Walsh and Goldrick, 1991). However, there is an exception, a network of psychotherapists who draw their conceptualising from Existentialism. The American, Irvin Yalom, a leading existential psychotherapist, maintains it 'gives an explicit place to the procedures which the majority of therapists employ implicitly' (Yalom, 1980). He provides a substantial reason for this subjugated discourse:

> The fear of death plays a major role in our internal experience: it haunts as does nothing else; it is a dark unsettling presence at the rim of consciousness ... The child at an early age is pervasively preoccupied with death, and his or her major developmental task is to deal with the terrifying fears of obliteration.

I worked recently with Sean, a 16-year-old, who has spent the last third of his life as a 'looked after' child in the care of the local authority. We had been working together for two years and were preparing for ending. He had made an audio recording for me of parts of the soundtrack of the film *The Sixth Sense* in which Bruce Willis plays a child therapist who encounters a child who can foresee the death of those around him. Sean had made the recording because he knew that I had not seen the film. He had also painstakingly transcribed whole sections of the script. He wanted me to know that the film had made him (nearly!) cry and to share the chilling fear of its content. Through the meticulous transcription of the text he 'externalized' his experiential difficulties and gained mastery over the death fear and our 'survival' after our work finished. The script provided the script.

The fear of annihilation, of non-being, is so embedded in our self experience that it cannot easily be given a voice or symbolic representation, though Sean was ingeniously able to find one. It is not sufficient to reduce it in the mechanistic language of biology to 'an instinct' as if that somehow 'explains' the experience. This submerged but integral part of our experience exercises influence over our psychic life if it remains, as Alfred Adler describes the unconscious, 'the not understood'. Yalom advances the radical hypothesis that death anxiety is the primary ground of psychosis and the dysfunction of mental health. 'Not understood', its capacity for disruption is immense.

> To cope with these fears we erect defences against death awareness, defences that are based on denial, that shape character structure and that, if maladaptive, result in clinical syndromes. In other words, psycho-pathology is the result of *ineffective modes of death transcendence* ... Death is a primordial source of anxiety and, as such, is the primary fount of psychotherapy. (Yalom, 1980)

In this, Yalom follows the American psychiatrist, Harold Searles, whose ideas were nearly contemporaneous with the Bateson group's work on schizophrenia. In a paper 'Schizophrenia and the Inevitability of Death' (1961), Searles took a slightly different perspective from the systemic double bind theory of Bateson's group, though there is scope for some synthesis of view:

> it is a matter rather of the patient's having become, and having long remained, schizophrenic (and reference here, of course, is to largely or wholly unconscious purposiveness) in order to avoid facing among other aspects of internal and external reality, the fact that life is finite.

On the basis of this hypothesis, finding a pharmacological cure for schizophrenia is as illusory as finding a cure for death, or reaching the horizon. The psychotherapist of whatever persuasion must, in Yalom's view, like everyone be actively existentially aware. This means tolerating the constant uncertainty of existence that comes from personal freedom and the termination of all things. Since every human context is pervaded by the changes imposed by transience (transition is the only change that never changes!) so no effective approach to psychotherapy should ignore this existential backcloth.

> Existence is inexorably free and, thus, uncertain. Cultural institutions and psychological constructs often obscure this state of affairs but confrontation with one's existential situation reminds one that paradigms are self-created, wafer-thin barriers against the pain of uncertainty. The mature therapist must in the existential theoretical approach as in any other, be able to tolerate this fundamental uncertainty. (Yalom, 1980)

Death, the tragic and our emotional life

The event of personal death is scripted into the human experience as certainly as the seasons and days and nights. Like the proverbial grit in an oyster, it is the catalyst in the search for meaning and for our being curious; our most profound emotional longings and thoughts; inspired and degrading actions; our relationships; our spiritual, aesthetic and scientific questing. Different cultures and religions have sought to give meaning and continuity to what is subjectively perceived as absurd, meaningless and the culmination of all futility. Just as we experience diffi- culty in perceiving the infinity of space, so we do the eternity of time. Yet we are beings who must face our relationship with the eternal, according to Kierkegaard. We are a long time dead! We cannot be certain our most cherished intrinsic relationships are likely to reconstitute; and this seems neither just, fair, rational nor explicable. Not surprisingly, the poet Dylan Thomas in the poem 'Do Not Go Gentle into That Good Night' (1951) urged an eloquent, raging, defiance of this human situation.

In the enantiodromic dynamic, our sense of concreteness, of continuity of somethingness is always faced with its opposite, the negation and nihila- tion of personal death. This is as much an interpersonal event as a personal one, for the ending of a life is as significant in its implicative effect for others as it is to the cessation of the person. So powerful are the emotions around death – our whole being is orientated in various levels of openness or avoidance to the possibility of dying – that it is difficult not to see it as the parent of all other bad and tragic experience. Loss (including health or function), separation and abandonment are the sibling experiences, the epiphenomena of the phenomenon of death; illness and violence are the pathways and the motions to rendering the invisible threat visible.

Death is an absolute. It is unchallenged as the event of moment in the hierarchy of human possibilities: the ending of all endings; the loss of all losses. The root of all trauma is not just the shock or the pain itself, which may be distressing enough, it is the confrontation with the death terror. Treatment of post-traumatic stress disorder does not always seem able to acknowledge this level of distress and treats the experience as if it were a technical matter of 'debriefing'. It is not surprising some research indicates mixed evidence for its value.

Yet clearly we are not defeated by death and developmentally we achieve effective *modes of death transcendence*. How is this done? Freud's belief was that it could be achieved through work, love and the acceptance of the finality of death (Freud, 1917) and not through Woody Allen's prescription, 'I shall not achieve immortality through my work, but by not dying'!

Death transcendence: existential realism and humour

The reality of death has been a theme throughout the history of philosophy. While much of it stressed the fear, the finality and inevitability, many philosophies have emphasised the freedom and completeness that comes from the acceptance of the inevitable. It may be the parent to tragedy, but it is equally the parent to wisdom. An existence without end would be intolerable. Death gives life its essence, as salt flavours food or the silver backing to glass transforms it into a mirror with reflecting qualities. Knowledge of our mortality is similarly the basis of our reflexivity and self-awareness. Pascal's *Pensées* (1670) articulates this in an eloquent statement of our capacity to think and of our 'emergence' into knowing reflection:

> Man is only a reed, the weakest in nature, but he is a thinking reed. There is no need for the whole universe to take up arms to crush him: a vapour, a drop of water is enough to kill him. But even if the universe were to crush him, man would still be nobler than his slayer, because he knows he is dying and the advantage the universe has over him. The universe knows none of this ... thus all our dignity consists in thought.

Though a rationalist, he was also aware of a deeper emotional intelligence we might now define as the unconscious: 'the heart has its reasons reason knows not'.

The Swiss psychiatrist Carl Jung regarded the unconscious as containing the means of death transcendence. In his BBC interview with John Freeman, on the *Face to Face* programme recorded in October 1959, he said:

> It is quite interesting to watch what the unconscious is doing with the fact that it is, apparently, threatened with the complete end. It disregards it. Life behaves as if it was going on ... It is better for old people to live on, to look forward to the next day as if he had to spend centuries. Then he lives properly. But, when he is afraid, if he doesn't look forward, he looks back, he petrifies ... he dies before his time. Of course it is obvious we are all going to die and this is the sad finale of everything, but nevertheless there is something in us that doesn't believe it apparently ... but this is merely a fact, a psychological fact.

Jung seems to propose an experiential paradox here: while not denying the finality of death, we operate as if it were not true and there were nothing to fear. This belief may be characterized as 'existential realism' in which the knowledge of death gives passion and activity to living. Our life is finite; it is not a resource to be squandered. Jung developed archetypal psychology in part to explain this psychological phenomenon. His ideas, like those of the existentialists, reintroduce beliefs about death that would have been part of the common currency of ideas among Greek and Roman philosophers and playwrights and oriental thinkers of the same period. Theirs are some of the earliest statements of existential realism.

At the end of *Oedipus the King* (Sophocles, c.429–420BC), the Chorus confronts the audience with the point of the tragedy, 'then learn that mortal man must always look to his ending'. Early philosophical movements like stoicism and epicurism stressed the awareness of death as a prerequisite of living properly. The Greek philosopher Socrates regarded philosophy itself to be a dialogue on death; the stoics thought similarly 'to philosophise is to prepare for death' (Cicero); 'no man enjoys the true taste of life but he who is willing and ready to quit it' (Seneca). Even early Christian thinkers saw the existential paradox: that to confront death is to confront life: 'It is only in the face of death that man's self is born' (St Augustine).

Buddhism, often described as an atheistic religion, is a disciplined spiritual way of living which places death awareness at the heart of the struggle for enlightenment and the means of becoming aware of all pretence and illusion. Existential realism provides the spiritual pathway for the seeker to achieve such transcendence (*The Dhammapada*, c.300BC):

> I have gone round in vain the cycles of many lives ever striving to find the builder of the house of life and death. How great is the sorrow of life that must die. ... Hidden in the mystery of consciousness, the mind, incorporeal, flies alone far away. Those who set their mind in harmony become free from the bonds of death.

A variation of this belief is echoed in existential psychotherapy but with a slightly different conclusion (Yalom, 1980):

> though the physicality of death destroys us, the idea of death saves us. Recognition of death contributes a sense of poignancy to life, provides a radical shift of life perspective and can transport one from one mode of living characterised by diversions, tranquillisation and petty anxieties to a more authentic one.

Humour is important in articulating and allowing cathartic release of the death anxiety. It can embrace the absurd, the flawed, the humiliating and the unjust and dissolve some of the tensions around them in ways that rationality cannot. Consider Woody Allen's famous paradox: 'I'm not afraid to die. I just don't want to be there when it happens' or Mark Twain's view (quoted in Enright, 1983): 'whoever has lived long enough to find out what life is, knows how deep a debt we owe to Adam, the first great benefactor of our race. He brought death into the world.' Family systems therapists such as Brian Cade (Cade, 2000) can use humour to powerful effect, following in the tradition of Carl Whitaker and John Weakland and Milton Erickson. Humour is a valuable tool in psychotherapy: it smoothes the formation of an effective working alliance with patients and detoxifies difficult issues.

Death transcendence: unconscious resources, art, culture and religion

Jung hypothesized that some part of our unconscious life contains the universal structure of a 'collective unconscious'. This processes experiences symbolically through archetypical forms, to which all human cultures have access and which assist creative living. This perspective sees 'the unconscious' as a resource, not necessarily a repository of fearful impulses. Archetypes, Jung insisted, are innate structures, like the universal ability for language. They are a kind of script but of universal roles, responses and relationships that may influence our psychological life. Louis Macneice's poem which begins this chapter can be understood in this way. The poem's central character finds himself connected to the archetype of his own father. For Jung, archetypes were spiritual, existential and biological imprints which, discovered through experience and awareness, lead to coherence and meaning. They provide some of the means of death transcendence. Stories, myths, art and dreams are all vehicles of the archetype's healing structures. Individuation, Jung's term for self-discovery, is itself a reflexive journey of the Self archetype.

Jung also thought religion was basically therapeutic. It provides a structure of belief, meaning, community, ritual (to mark life-cycle transitions) and alleviation of suffering. In existential terms, world religions do not shun or deny the presence of death, but offer beliefs about the mystery. Most religions have their stories about the purpose of death, and all seek to combat intrusive thoughts of nihilation and absurdity. Some are optimistic, and encourage a 'better character'. Christianity has often used its narratives shamelessly as a means of moral enforcement, even seemingly, to extol the virtues of death over life – 'pie in the sky when you die', as it was popularly known. For societies where death rates were high and life expectancy low, these narratives may have been existentially comforting. In the West, better public health and warfare have made these accounts seem inadequate placebos to the growing sceptical audience. Here, postmodern secular ideas, mostly based on a kind of individualistic hedonism and personal lifestyle choice, which takes the boundary of death as an injunction to 'live life to the full while we still have it', have largely replaced the dread of a judged unpleasant afterlife.

The mystical and contemplative traditions in the major world religions direct the seeker to the ecstasy of divine love; the inner peaceful acceptance of self; to silence, stillness and an active union with emptiness of thought (of the 'nada', in fact), as a goal of mental attention. Indeed, meditational practice, at one level, enacts the state of preparedness for death that the 'best deaths' manage. Anger, the 'raging against the dying of the light', though very natural, is not considered beneficial in these traditions, though it clearly spoke to some of the self-destructive elements in Dylan Thomas. Art, poetry, drama, music and the creative arts, like humour, help to give voice to the unbearable darkness of being and not only render it more bearable, but raise up the joy of creativity, spontaneity and the celebration of living.

Death transcendence: attachment and the human family

Of all the social structures existing to mediate the finality of personal death, 'the family' is the most persistent and accomplished. It is difficult to maintain that this is its function, for in no sense is the family a purposive creation, nor is it a singular, homogenous entity. The family is a social arrangement for nurturing children and provide caregiving across at least two generations in a unit of shared identity and identification. Yet enduring and evolving, it is the single most common means of death transcendence. Though the person is mortal; the family as a system and an identifiable group is somehow immortal. The growth industry of genealogical research gives some evidence of this, while other cultural traditions keep their family stories alive through transmitted oral history. The impetus is the profound curiosity rooted in the family's existential significance and validity. This is not to idealize families nor family life, but to state one of its deeply rooted strengths as a defence against annihilation.

The form and pattern the family takes is culturally and historically specific, and so is liable to change over time with globalization, different images of family life style and migration. The transformed attitude to divorce in Britain has created a new nexus of extended family relationships through recreated family structures. The development of same sex parenting partnerships is a significant change as part of this revolution. Replication of family life through fostering and adoption has been a vital instrument of social policy in seeking to repair, ironically, the many adverse effects that family life can have on the development of secure identity in children.

The family therefore is an existentially constituted unit which seeks to surmount the human life-cycle as a surfer rides the waves. The emotions to do with the sorrow of disaster, loss and the tragic enforce in a circular way those of the joy of belonging and participating. It is a human crucible, the drama workshop, in which all most basic and significant human emotions and sense of the secure are melded and exchanged.

> Emotion provides the thread and colour in the tapestry of family life. The full range of every experience is felt most profoundly within family relationships: bliss, contentment, sexual ecstasy, loyalty, remorse, loneliness, frustration, boredom, fear, murderous rage and so on. Feelings provide the impetus for staying together and for leaving. They energise relationships. (Byng Hall, 1982b)

The heart's reasons of which reason knows not are developed and experienced over time most emphatically in the family. The Freudian interpretation of the Oepidus story subordinates the most interesting and obvious conclusion of the 'family romance' – that family life is always potent with passion, anxiety and the mediation of death. Family therapists have helped to restore the multi-perspective dynamic inherent in the myth and restored the family's therapeutic potential and resourcefulness and not, as Freud seemed to emphasise, its therapeutic destructiveness.

Through its narratives, traditions and its archetypical embodiment, the family is imperishable. This is the greatest transcendence of all: the endurance beyond death; the coalesced triumph of human, biological, cultural and existential accomplishment. Attachment is the instrument of this triumph. It is important not only for itself but because of the security it provides against that terror of annihilation and the 'nada'. This is what makes the child secure and able to develop defences against dying. The quality of attachment is absolute because death is absolute:

> attachment behaviour is any form of behaviour that results in a person attaining or maintaining proximity to some other clearly identified individual who is conceived as better able to cope with the world. It is most obvious whenever the person is frightened fatigued or sick and is assuaged by comforting and caregiving ... whilst ... at its most obvious in early childhood, it can be observed throughout the life cycle (Bowlby, 1988).

Within the universality of attachment, there are many archetypal forms of human love and care for which the family is the matrix: maternal love, paternal love, filial love, fraternal and sororal love, gerontic love, ancestral love and love that generalizes into empathy and communal care through the process Alfred Adler defined as 'social interest' (Hills, 1999). Birth, the embodiment of new creation, is the biological and experiential corrective to death – the instinctive and emotional antidote to the nullification of being. The full awareness that loving another being is the more intense and piquant because it happens in the face of non-being, is at the heart of familial love and attachment.

Whether a family is created through biological, legal, situational and recreated means matters little compared with its potentiality for attachment. The social arrangement called 'the family' exists significantly therefore as an existential defence. It has a deep resilience against political, social, historical or natural acts of catastrophe or oppression, from slavery to the holocaust, which serves to affirm itself as both defence and defiance against the absurdity of death and the depredation of social and political oppression. Social policy-makers rarely seem to conceptualize it in such a way but are more prone to attack it as a conservative force, resistant to political ideology, or readily embrace it to save the state the cost of social care. If death is that which dare not speak its name, it is unsurprising that the family, as a primary existential defence against it, is likewise unstated.

Death is as much a family event as birth. As well as marking the life-cycle changes, it defines the family. It is through our family links and networks that we are somehow preserved and have influence for a time after our personal existence has ceased. Despite the plainer postmodern death rituals of biodegradable cardboard coffins and scattering ashes, etc., personal identity is preserved, as it always has been, through the remembrance of friends and colleagues but mostly the family. As W.H. Auden said on the death of his fellow poet, W.B. Yeats, 'He became his followers', so in a sense most deceased 'become their family'.

Individuals remain alive in these family memories long after they have died, though, of course, how they are remembered is often connected with what they did and how they were in life. It secures a kind of resurrection, and is the beginning of the creation of family myth, legend and script. Archie Smith, an African American family therapist and Baptist pastor, put it with simple eloquence when describing the beliefs of Black American churches (Smith, 2001): 'There are the living; the living dead; and the dead dead. The living dead are alive for as long as there are still others left to remember them, then they become the dead dead.'

Family scripts

Bowlby (1988) maintained that besides providing a depth of assurance, comfort and security through attachment, much of the family interactional pattern is also internalized and a child constructs an active model of his parents and their interaction:

> subsequently the model of himself that the child builds reflects also the images his parents have of him, images that are communicated not only by how each treats him, but by what each says to him ... once built ... are so taken for granted that they come to operate at an unconscious level.

This experience is the heart of the metaphor of the family script. Not only does attachment define the pattern of caregiving and nurturing but on this reading it provides the experiential framework, the enscriptment for the totality of the cognitive, emotional, acting, interacting and storytelling repertoire, for both family and person. This is how the community of internalized others finds its expression, through being both observer and actor of 'the script', which is drafted and redrafted over time and engaged through osmosis and mimesis. While Bowlby's description of attachment seems to centre on the relationship between child and parent, it clearly operates between different combinations of cross and intergenerational relationships.

Where there is little attachment or neglect or abuse, the script may be one of void, emptiness and the existential experience of the 'nada'. John Byng-Hall's main description of script analysis is to point to the enantrio-dromic process of correction-replication, enacted overtly or uncon-sciously. Helping to find a coherent narrative form is to invite the possibility of transcending the emotional thrall of the script.

This process can be seen at many levels in Louis Macneice's poem, 'The Truisms' (1988). Clearly based on the parable of the prodigal son, the subject of the poem leaves home, rejecting the family's beliefs. This is the corrective tendency in the script, though there is no stated description about any replacement – it seems to be a quest for different experiences. In time, through the same experiences, he completes the circularity of his journey back to his roots: 'something told him the way to behave. He raised his hand and blessed his home.' In the enantriodromic response to the script, this is the correction to the correction – the replicative element. The 'truisms' are not defined and can symbolize the wisdom of the family, the activation of archetypical role, identification, the transcendence over death, the life-stage transition from father to son, as well as a vivid descrip-tion of the 'emergence' into consciousness of the influence of family script and attachment.

The threat of the tragic particularly activates family scripts. The gestalt of the script may replicate a paralysis of thought or feeling. Alternatively, it may impart wisdom or alarm, orientating family members' thinking and behaving towards the threats to their continuity. Scripts that are existen-tially based around death as a real possibility that can be thought about, are likely to better orientate the family. Existential realism, as we have seen, will produce a better sense of transcendence. Much of the basic work of therapy is to help the family produce a better account of their situation and examine the patterns, assumptions, replications, corrections which have developed about tragic narratives. So the process moves, like

Macneice's subject, from unexamined response to deeper affiliation and connection.

The experience of death often deepens and strengthens what was present in life, from the sense of belonging and attachment to family structure and heritage. Human existence can be encountered with zest, interest and commitment. Living fully does not have to mean fearing death, though respecting it. This experience can be embodied in the family script; when it is not, helping the family to seek to rewrite it is a central challenge of the therapy.

Four existential fragments of family scripts

1 The Sharp family

The family had been for family therapy some six years before Margaret's referral for individual work, but this had ended abruptly because her husband, Terrence, had withdrawn, objecting to the presence of a team and a one-way screen. Though described as a skilful amateur artist, family members complained that he was cold 'control freak'. He was said to have frequent outbursts at family gatherings, disappointed with his children's careers and academic achievements, comparing them adversely to himself. He was particularly dismissive towards Belinda who had been diagnosed with manic-depression (bi-polar affective disorder) in her twenties and who had been hospitalized on several occasions. The antithesis of her father's controlled, socially conventional personality, she revelled in displays of rebellion and defiance that frequently bordered on the self-destructive. In her late thirties, close to completing a social care course, she suddenly dropped out of her studies, got admitted and then discharged herself from a psychiatric unit and lived as a virtual recluse with her mother.

Several years before this, Margaret had entered a very intense period of individual psychotherapy, based on a systemic perspective, in which she'd closely examined her whole life and the points of distress: the sexually abusive father of the Liverpool family where she had been evacuated as a child; the departure of her own father for another woman after the war; his imprisonment for embezzlement; her care of her younger sister and mentally ill brother during her mother's acute bouts of depression; and her mother's subsequent suicide when Margaret was pregnant with her first child, just after her marriage. For Margaret, marriage had been an escape, security with a husband who

> put me on a pedestal and since no one had ever put me there before, I was only too happy to remain there. For me he was my romantic hero. I little knew how much damage he would later do to our children and me.

In the early years of the marriage each had felt satisfied; both had conventional expectations of each other and their relationship, and were pleased when Margaret became pregnant with Rosalyn. Her husband, Terrence, was an only child who was said to have a rather formal relationship with his mother who, in return, idolized him. He had achieved one of his goals in starting a family and fulfilling himself as a man, as provider. Within her birth family, Margaret, as the eldest sibling, had always taken the role of the 'little mother'. In her family of creation, through her husband's attentiveness and secure high income, she felt that she was now 'being cared for', and she was able to withstand some of the immediate effects of her mother's suicide.

At an emotional level, Margaret had resolved that she would always be a reliable source of attachment for her children. She had grown up in considerable hardship, experiencing her mother's frequent change of moods and acute depression, and the prevailing family belief that at any stage she might commit suicide. Thus, as part of her corrective script, she had secured a reliable partner whose income helped provide a contained space in which she had four children.

Her pregnancies were uncomplicated. However, following the birth of Cynthia, Belinda, their second child, became increasingly anxiously attached. She would produce tantrums and defiant behaviour well beyond the capacity of the parents to manage or contain, and evolved various signs of anxiety phobia and withdrawal. This pattern, once established, created a structural realignment, in which Terrence became disengaged and Margaret enmeshed, while the three other siblings increasingly experiencing their mother as being more available to their sister than themselves. The parents quarrelled with increasing passion and a growing shared dislike. No assessment was ever sought for Belinda or the family's distress, and the pattern continued through adolescence into young adulthood, when Belinda was treated for bi-polar affective disorder, often through hospitalization. She was seen by the family as loud, aggressive, unpredictable, rarely took her medication, and would increasingly engender her father's cold anger and emotional rejection. He had withdrawn increasingly from his wife, and would bully and criticize the children during their adolescence, and especially Belinda. The more ill Belinda became, the more Margaret found herself drawn into the replicative script of caretaking a suicidal family member and the more her husband's experiential pathway replicated her father's. He had affairs and eventually left her for another woman.

Belinda struggled hard to locate herself in a career, and was accepted for training as a social care worker. This went well until her final placement. She became increasingly depressed, suicidal, and was twice hospitalized. She made two serious suicide attempts, one, by attempting to hang herself, and the second walking on an electrified railway line. The more suicidal she became, the more enmeshed was the relationship with Margaret. As a result, she refused to be hospitalized and grew increasingly reliant on her mother with whom she lived; the more perturbed she became, the more intensely her mother sought to prevent her from killing herself. However, at the age of 38, one afternoon while her mother was asleep, Belinda hanged herself from the tree in the garden. In a brief suicide note, she apologized to her mother and the family, saying that she believed that her earlier suicide attempt had caused her brain damage, and death was the only way she would find peace.

Her mother was devastated, full of self-reproach, and returned for further therapy, microscopically examining her role in what had transpired. She came to understand from criticism from her children and her own examination that she believed she should have left the children's father earlier, and had failed to protect them from his emotional assaults on them. Looking over Belinda's psychiatric case notes that she requested after her death, she realized with utter clarity just how destructive Belinda had found family relationships and her father's disapproval. Margaret's corrective-scripted attempt to preserve family unity and her availability to her children had been paradoxical in its outcome. From the bleakness of these discoveries she struggled to make peace with herself, her children and Belinda. Terrence, however, dismissed any attempt, notably from the son William, to make him feel responsible in any way for Belinda's suicide and immersed himself in his second family.

There are many more rich undercurrents in this family drama than this brief narrative can include. It is impossible not to see the tragic working through of the interweaving of a number of scripts, and how, paradoxically, the attempt to correct resulted in the replication of the tragedy. There are many 'might have beens'. Like the process of Greek tragedy, death was scripted both as a catastrophe to be avoided, a means of release from intolerable experience and a enantriodromic family pattern of too much and too little responsibility for helping to alleviate the distress of other members of the family. Sometimes the existential pattern is so deeply set it eludes the best attempts to challenge it, for it is not given to psychotherapists to play providence or provide the *deus ex machina*.

2 Judy and Donald Palmer

Judy is in her late forties and married to Donald, who is slightly older. He's a quiet, thin, asthmatic man who has been running a successful agricultural retail firm for the last 18 years. They have been married for 20 years and have two children, a son Jack, 18, who works in London, and a daughter Cecile, 14, who is at boarding school. They describe their marriage as extremely happy for the first 15 years (rating it happy 80 per cent of the time). However, now their marriage is in some crisis with Judy convinced that Donald has been having an affair with Susie, his secretary, for the past three years. During the session, she produces detailed circumstantial evidence of this: his buying Susie flowers; their being seen dining out together; her affectionate Christmas card thanking him for his present; his ringing her immediately after the Millennium. He steadfastly denies he is having an affair, though agrees that he has crossed the boundary from a professional to an intense personal friendship and involvement. They agree, eventually, that though the relationship with Susie may not have been sexual it was inappropriately intimate in every other way and had reduced the affection between them. Judy is very angry and during the joint sessions attacks him ferociously and remorselessly. His reasoned counter arguments intensify her suspicion and hostility; these repetitious, set-piece arguments happen outside the session and drove the couple into seeking therapy in the first place. Their children just stand aside and shrug their shoulders in a 'there's Mum and Dad at it again' resigned way. They speak together of never having disagreements in the first 15 years of the relationship and not managing agreements in the last three.

Looking at their family scripts it becomes apparent that for Judy, the experience at the age of seven of her attentive father's sudden death in a road traffic accident has remained a defining experience. For a time she was separated from her three other siblings to live with the extended family. She watched her mother struggle to reunite the family and bring up all four children alone. She chose a partner like Don whose reliability and dependability were absolute. They evolved a pattern, unique among their friends, that if ever they disagreed, she would ring immediately to apologize automatically, adding: 'If anything happens to me suddenly I want you to know I'm sorry.' It was part of their 'making up' ritual and the recent disagreement over Donald's relationship with the secretary was therefore radically different – no one was backing down. Though he terminated the employment of his secretary, Judy reacted by asserting her independence, going out with single women friends to nightclubs, driving Donald into reciprocal jealousy. The game is at deuce and they know it. This change has been uncomfortable for them both, but they want to retrieve the relationship. They also know they have to develop a very different script and they are working on it.

3 Josie Andrews

Josie is a 29-year-old nurse working with seriously ill patients. She is bedevilled by feelings of depression when she is not at work and only comes alive at work where she is highly attuned, caring and responsive to her patients. On a number of occasions she has identified intuitively health and psychological difficulties that her patients are suffering from and this understanding has helped to shorten their distress. Josie, however, frequently feels suicidal and made two serious attempts. As a student she had a history of self-cutting, which culminated in her first suicide attempt by overdose. The junior doctor attending her at the time told her mockingly, 'Well, we won't be trying that again, will we?' She was incensed at this remark and had some paradoxical satisfaction, in proving him wrong in her second overdose several months later, but little else.

She spoke of growing up in the shadow of her mother's manic depression and worked hard to make herself helpful to her mother and yet invisible, lest she incurred her mother's violent rages. The father of her friend interfered with her sexually when she was six. Her quarrelsome parents separated and there was a bitter custody dispute. Her father only ever showed interest in her older sister, and he subsequently left Britain to work in America. Her mother and sister would argue ferociously and she resolved to remain emotionally unresponsive so as not to antagonize her mother unnecessarily. The third generation of a strict fundamentalist sect, though non-churchgoing, Josie as a child had strongly identified with the life-script and example of Jesus. She constructed a profound belief in which she wished to sacrifice her own life to save her mother's. In certain moods, her mother made it clear to them she regretted the birth of Josie and her sister.

On the first sessions she said that her sense of reality suddenly came to an end at the age of 14 as she was walking through her home town in Surrey. Nothing, she said, suddenly seemed real and she lost any sense of who she was. She responded well to a few teachers who encouraged her and won some prizes at secondary school for her writing. At 14, however, one of the teachers who encouraged her, and who was advanced in her pregnancy, was killed in a road traffic accident; her mother prevented her from attending the funeral on the basis that the death had nothing to do with her, and would only distress her. Her rage towards her mother is palpable but denied. At that moment, death became a means of escape, defiance and ultimate sacrifice and nullification of her being. Like many self-harmers, she found emotional release from drawing blood. Therapeutic work, then, is to help her explore the meaning that death holds for her and the thrall of sacrifice. She cannot express hatred towards her parents, for that, she believes, would be weakness and personal moral failure, nor can she forgive either.

4 Stuart McKay

Stuart is a 26-year-old who was born with a heart defect. He was active as a child, playing soccer which he loved. In junior school he became conscious of hesitating on certain words and would go out of his way to alter sentences and words to avoid revealing his speech hesitation. At the same time his father who had a serious drink problem would sometimes drive him to football matches under the influence, colliding with the pavement and parked cars. He would often fall asleep and miss Stuart's match. At the age of 12 Stuart had a mild operation to stimulate the function of the aorta valve in his heart. At first it seemed a success, but within 18 hours, the consultant told Stuart that he would need open heart surgery, he should give up sport and any idea of a career in the RAF. He thought briefly of jumping to his death through the hospital window but dismissed the idea as an absurd response to his desired health.

At 15 he had the open heart surgery, made a good recovery and was encouraged by hospital staff to act as counsellor to other children on the ward to help them combat their fears. This he did several times willingly, but a 14-year-old, whom he helped to reassure, did not recover. Stuart feels an enduring sense of guilt and feels unable to face the follow-up operation he needs himself. 'The trouble is everyone thinks I'm confident but I'm afraid to die. I don't believe there's anything afterwards and you don't come back, even as a snail.' He is more worried about his speech hesitancy than his heart condition, for he believes it is holding back his life. He now gets his father to speak on the phone for him even though he used to make announcements on a public address system in one of his jobs. His partner wants to have children, but Stuart is deeply confused about this and cannot see a future for himself. During therapy he said suddenly, 'I think I worry about my speech to take my mind off thinking about my heart.' He asked if his father could join the therapy and his father agreed to do so. His father spoke openly about his own experience of 'nada' through his alcoholism, and from which with therapeutic help he eventually emerged. Three sessions later Stuart felt able to actively face and agree to the necessary corrective heart surgery he had been resisting.

Conclusion

Death is a difficult subject to examine. Though it is a natural process that is part of the whole integrity of human existence, it is an absolute defining life event through the impermeable boundary it sets and the mystery which lies beyond it. The human family, though developed in many different forms and shapes, nonetheless, is the single greatest human attempt to seek transcendence of death with the celebration of shared being, passing on culture, identity, love, care, attachment and a sense of the good; to combat the threatening nullification of death, the impingement of the absurd and nothingness of 'nada'. It is both a human defence against death, but needs itself to find defences from within to renew its resilience and shared sense of belonging which the finality of loss attacks fundamentally.

Family scripts provide part of the attachment architecture, the emotional, behavioural and cognitive structures which imbue relationships with meaning and value. These are, however, constructs and have to be revisited and revised in the face of challenges to their adequacy which go to the depth of the shared human family experience. The deepest and worse existential encounter is that with death and families may need most help to rescript the 'reasons of the heart which reason knows not' which arise from the existential abyss and vertiginous state which death may present.

Mourning and loss are always a family event, and each member's reaction may be different: what happens or what fails to happen; what emotional life is expressed or remains dormant; what is thought about together; what stories are told to whom about what, and how they are amended – this is at the heart of family process. Like Jung's notion of archetypical psychology, family scripts often operate as an invisible influence.

However, existence itself provides the material for the script and this existential ground should hold the therapist's attention, to have a full appreciation of the working dynamic of each family script. It is as if life itself, the context of contexts, is so vast and common an experience that it should not be thought about. Nothing can be further from the truth.

It is through our centredness in existence that we are made members of the community of therapeutic voices. Therapy may have no greater contribution to the mystery of existence and successful living than any other discipline. What it can identify, through human curiosity and an attentive being with others, is where to look and how to look through the glass lightly.

John Hills trained as a social worker at the University of Kent in 1972 and worked at the Lenworth Child and Family Psychiatry Clinic in Ashford Kent. He completed his training in family therapy and live supervision at the Tavistock Clinic in London in 1984 and has worked as a systemic psychotherapist in the NHS in Canterbury since 1988, first in child and family mental health, and in 1991 at the Cossington Road, Adult Psychotherapy Clinic. He also works independently. In 1989 he was the founding editor of Context, *a news magazine for members of the Association for Family Therapy and Systemic Practice and continues as its general editor. He has been a member of the board of AFT since 1983. He is a course tutor on the intermediate family systemic training course at the Tavistock Clinic. A Quaker, his other major interest is singing and playing rhythm and blues with the Reunion Blues Band.*

References

Al-Issa I (1995) Handbook of Culture and Mental Illness. Madison, CT: International Universities Press.

Andersen T (1987) The reflecting team: dialogue and meta-dialogue in clinical work, Family Process 26: 415–28.

Asen KE, Jenkins H (1992) Family therapy without the family: a framework for systemic practice, Journal of Family Therapy 14: 1–14.

Asen KE, Tomson P (1987) Family Solutions in Family Practice. Lancaster: Quay.

Bakhtin M (1981) Dialogic Imagination: Four Essays. Austin, TX: University of Texas Press.

Barrett W (1961) Irrational Man: A Study in Existential Philosophy. London: Heinemann.

Bell JE (1951) Family Group Therapy. Public Health Monograph, No. 64. US Dept of Health, Education and Welfare.

Boal A (1992) Games for Actors and Non-Actors. Transl. A Jackson. London: Routledge.

Boal A (1998) Theatre of the Oppressed. London: Pluto Press.

Boscolo L, Bertrando P (1996) Systemic Therapy with Individuals. London: Karnac Books.

Boscolo L, Cecchin G, Selvini Palazzoli M, Prata G (1980) Hypothesising, circularity, neutrality, Family Process 19(1): 3–12.

Boszormenyi-Nagy Spark I (1973) Invisible Loyalties. London: Harper & Row.

Bowlby J (1949) The study and reduction of group tensions in the family. Human Relations 2: 123.

Bowlby J (1953) Child Care and the Growth of Love. London: Penguin Books.

Bowlby J (1969) Attachment. London: Hogarth Press.

Bowlby J. (1988) A Secure Base: Clinical Applications of Attachment Theory. London: Routledge.

Boyd JH, Weissman MM (1982) Epidemiology of affective disorder: a re-examination and future directions, Archives of General Psychiatry 38(9), September.

Boyd-Franklin N (1989) Black Families in Therapy. New York: Guilford Press.

Brecht B (1976) Poems 1913–1956. Eds J Willett, R Manheim. London: Methuen.

Brecht B (1980) Mother Courage and Her Children. Transl. J Willett, eds J Willett, R Manheim. London & New York, Methuen.

Brown J (1997) Circular questioning: an introductory guide, Australian and New Zealand Journal of Family Therapy 18(2).

Bruggen P, Byng-Hall J, Pitt-Aikens T (1971) The reason for admission as a focus of work on an adolescent unit, British Journal of Psychiatry 122: 319–29.

Byng-Hall J (1973) Family myths used as defence in conjoint family therapy, British Journal of Psychology 46: 239–50.

Byng-Hall J (1979) Re-editing family mythology during family therapy, Journal of Family Therapy 1(2): 103–16.

Byng-Hall J (1980) Symptom bearer as marital distance regulator: clinical implications, Family Process 19: 355–65.

Byng-Hall J (1982a) Family legends: their significance for the family therapist. In A Bentovim et al. (eds), Family Therapy: Complementary Frameworks of Theory and Practice. Vol. 2. London: Academic Press.

Byng-Hall J (1982b) Dysfunction of feeling: experiential life of the family. In A Bentovim, G Gorell Barnes, A Cooklin (eds), Family Therapy: Complementary Frameworks of Theory and Practice. Vol. 2. London, Academic Press.

Byng-Hall J (1985) The family script: a useful bridge between theory and practice, Journal of Family Therapy 7: 301–5.

Byng-Hall J (1986) Family scripts: a concept which can bridge child psychotherapy and family therapy thinking, Journal of Child Psychotherapy 12(1): 3-13.

Byng-Hall J (1991) An appreciation of John Bowlby: his significance for family therapy. Journal of Family Therapy 13(1): 5–16.

Byng-Hall J (1995a) Creating a secure family base: some implications of attachment theory for family therapy, Family Process 19: 45–57.

Byng-Hall J (1995b) Rewriting Family Scripts: Improvisation and Systems Change. London: Guildford Publications.

Byng-Hall J (1997) Toward a coherent story in illness and loss. In R Papodopoulos, J Byng-Hall, Multiple Voices: Narratives in Systemic Family Psychotherapy. London: Duckworth.

Byng-Hall J (1998) Evolving ideas about narrative: re-editing the re-editing of family mythology, Journal of Family Therapy 20: 133–42.

Byng-Hall J (1999a) Creating a coherent story in family therapy. In G Roberts, J Holmes (eds), Narrative Approaches in Psychiatry and Psychotherapy. Oxford: Oxford University Press.

Byng-Hall J (1999b) Family and couple therapy: toward greater security. In J Cassidy, PR Shaver (eds), Handbook of Attachment: Theory, Research and Clinical Applications. New York: Guilford Press.

Byng-Hall J, Bruggen P (1974) Family admission decisions as a therapeutic tool, Family Process 13: 443–59.

Cade B (2000) The Interactional View: The Use of Humour and the Unpredictable in Brief Therapy. PO Box 386, Eastwood NSW, 2122.

Campbell D (1999) Family therapy and beyond: where is the Milan systemic approach today?, Child Psychology and Psychiatry Review. Vol 4, No. 2. pp. 76–84.

Campbell D (2000) Socially Constructed Organisation. London: Karnac Books.

Campbell D, Draper R (eds) (1985) Applications of Systemic Family Therapy: The Milan Approach. London, Grune & Stratton.

Campbell D, Draper R, Crutchley E (1991) The Milan systemic approach to family therapy. In A Gurman, D Kniskern (eds), Handbook of Family Therapy. Vol. 2. New York: Brunner/Mazel.

Chekhov A [1904] The Cherry Orchard. Transl. H Rappaport. London: Faber & Faber (1978).

Corey G, Bitter JR (1996) Family systems therapy. In G Corey (ed.), Theory and Practice of Counseling and Psychotherapy. 5th edn. Pacific Grove, California: Brooks/Cole.

Cronen V, Johnson K, Lannaman J (1982) Paradoxes, double binds and reflexive loops: an alternative theoretical perspective, Family Process 21: 91–112.

Cronen V, Pearce WB (1985) Towards an explanation of how the Milan method works. In D Campbell, R Draper (eds), Applications of Systemic Family Therapy: the Milan Approach. London: Grune & Stratton.

The Dhammapada [c. 300 BC] Authors unknown (1975) London: Penguin Books

Enright DJ (ed.) (1983) The Oxford Book of Death. Oxford: Oxford University Press.

Esslin M (1984) Brecht: A Choice of Evils. London & New York: Methuen.

Eyre R (2001) Keynote address, Theatre 2001 conference. London.

Fadiman A (1997) The Spirit Catches You and You Fall Down. New York: Noonday Press.

Flaskas C (1993) On the project of using psychoanalytic ideas in systemic therapy, Australian and New Zealand Journal of Family Therapy 14(1): 9–15.

Flaskas C (1999) Limits and possibilities of the postmodern narrative self, Australian and New Zealand Journal of Family Therapy 20(1): 20–7.

Fleuridas C et al. (1986) The evolution of circular questions: training family therapists, Journal of Marital and Family Therapy 12(2).

Fredman G (1997) Death talk. London: Karnac Books.

Freud S. (1916) Introductory Lectures on Psychoanalysis. London: Penguin (1974).

Freud S (1917) Melancholy and Mourning: The Complete Psychological Works of Sigmund Freud. Vol 13. London: Hogarth Press.

Greenhalgh T, Hurwitz B (1998) Narrative Based Medicine. London: BMJ Books.

Handler L (1972) The amelioration of nightmares in children, Psychotherapy: Theory, Research and Practice 54–6.

Hills J (1999) Socialist constructionism: the revolution of re-inventing the wheel, Context 45.

Hingley R (1966) Chekhov. London: Unwin.

Hoffman L (1981) Foundations of Family Therapy. New York: Basic Books.

Huygen FJA (1978) Family Medicine: The Medical Life History of Families. Nijmegan: Dekker & Van De Vegt.

Jones E, Asen E (2000) Systemic Couple Therapy and Depression. London: Karnac.

Jones P (1996) Drama as Therapy; Theatre as Living. London: Routledge.

Kaftanzi V (1997) From Ancient Chorus to the Reflecting Team. Transl. K. Vevas. Presentation at the 25th Anniversary of the Milan School of Systemic Therapy.

Kierkegaard S (1843) Fear and Trembling and Sickness unto Death. Transl. Lowrie. Princeton, NJ: Princeton Press (1974).

Kitzinger C, Wilkinson S (1996) Theorizing representing the other. In S Wilkinson, C Kitzinger (eds), Representing the Other: A Feminism and Psychology Reader. London: Sage.

Kleinman A (1988) The Illness Narratives. New York: Basic Books.

Koestler A (1975) The Ghost in the Machine. London: Picador.

Koestler A (1980) Bricks to Babel. London: Picador.

Larner G (1999) The 'unfashionable' John Byng-Hall: narrative, myths and attachment, Australian and New Zealand Journal of Family Therapy 20(1): 34–9.

Leff J et al. (2000) The London depression intervention trial, British Journal of Psychiatry 177: 95–100.

McDaniels et al. (1997) The Shared Experience of Illness: Stories from Patients, Families and Their Therapists. New York: Basic Books.

McGoldrick M (1982) Through the looking glass: supervision of a trainee's 'trigger' family. In R Whiffen, J Byng-Hall (eds), Family Therapy Supervision: Recent Developments in Practice. London: Academic Press.

MacKinnon L, Miller D (1987) The new epistemology and the Milan approach: feminist and sociopolitical considerations, Journal of Marital and Family Therapy 13: 139–55.

Macneice L (1988) Selected Poems. London: Faber.

Macquarrie J (1980) Existentialism. London: Penguin Books.

Magagna J (1987) Three years of infant observation with Mrs Bick, Journal of Child Psychotherapy 13(1).

Main M, Kaplan N, Cassidy J (1985) Security in infancy, childhood, and adulthood: a move to the level of representation. In I Bretherton, E Waters (eds), Monograph of the Society for Research in Child Development, Serial No. 209, 50, Nos 1–2. The University of Chicago Press.

Martin F, Knight J (1962) Joint interviews as part of intake procedure in a child psychiatric clinic, Journal of Child Psychology and Psychiatry 3: 17–26.

Miller A (1956) The family in modern drama, Atlantic Monthly.

Miller A [1949] Death of a Salesman. In Plays: One. London: Methuen (1988).

Minghella A (1993) Presentation extract MA course in Playwriting. University of Birmingham.

Minuchin S (1974) Families and Family Therapy. Boston, MA: Harvard University Press; London: Tavistock.

Minuchin S, Fishman H (1981) Family Therapy Techniques. Boston, MA: Harvard University Press.

Moreno J (1946, 1959) Psychodrama. Vols 1 & 2. New York: Beacon House.

National Statistics (2000) Key Health Statistics from General Practice 1998. London.

Pascal B (1670) Pensées. London, Penguin Books (1995).

Pearce J, Cronin V (1980) Communication, Action and Meaning: The Creation of Social Realities. New York: Praeger.

Pearlman A (1992) Lecture: Modern European Drama. University of Kent, Canterbury.

Pinter H [1965] The Homecoming. Plays Three. London: Eyre Methuen (1978).

Rame F, Fo D (1990) The Open Couple. Transl. S Hood. London: Methuen.

Rangell L (1950) A treatment of nightmares in a seven-year-old boy, Psychoanalytic Study of the Child 5: 358–85.

Regier et al. (1988) Psychiatric Disorders in the Community. Epidemiological Catchment Area Study. From Hales R, Frances A (eds) American Psychiatric Association Annual Review. Vol 6, pp. 610–624. Washington DC: American Psychiatric Press Inc.

Rolland J (1994) Working with illness: clinicians' personal and interface issues, Family Systems Medicine 12(4).

Rycroft P, Perlesz A (2001) Speaking the unspeakable: reclaiming grief and loss in family life, Australian and New Zealand Journal of Family Therapy 22(1): 57–65.

Sampson E (1993) Celebrating the Other. Boulder, CO: Westview Press.

Searles H (1961) Schizophrenia and the inevitability of death, Psychiatric Quarterly 35: 631–55.

Selvini Palazzoli M et al. (1974) The treatment of children through brief therapy of their parents, Family Process 13: 429–42.

Selvini Palazzoli M et al. (1978) Paradox and Counterparadox. New York: Aronson.

Selvini Palazzoli M et al. (1980) Hypothesizing-circularity-neutrality: three guidelines for the conductor of the session, Family Process 19: 3–12.

Smith A (2001) The Spiritual Beliefs of African-American Churches. Presentation, 10 January, Tavistock Clinic, London.

Sophocles (c. 429–420BC) The Theban Plays. Transl. EF Watling. London: Penguin (1959).

Skynner ARC (1976) One Flesh: Separate Person. London: Constable.

Tomm K (1984a) One perspective on the Milan systemic approach: Part 1. Overview of development, theory and practice, Journal of Marital and Family Therapy 10: 113–25.

Tomm K (1984b) One perspective on the Milan systemic approach: Part 2. Description of session format, interviewing style and interventions, Journal of Marital and Family Therapy 10: 253–71.

Tomm K (1988) Interventive interviewing: Part 111. Intending to ask lineal, circular, strategic or reflexive questions, Family Process 27: 1–16.

Thomas D (1951) Collected Poems 1934–1953. London: Dent (1997).

Trevarthen C (1979) Communication and co-operation in early infancy: a description of primary intersubjectivity. In M Bullowa (ed.), Before Speech: The Beginning of Interpersonal Communication. Cambridge: Cambridge University Press.

Walsh F, McGoldrick M (eds) (1991) Living Beyond Loss: Death in the Family. New York: Norton.

Whiffen R, Byng-Hall J (eds) (1982) Family Therapy Supervision: Recent Developments in Practice. London: Academic Press; New York & San Francisco, Grune and Stratton.

White M (1989) Selected Papers. Adelaide: Dulwich Centre Publications.

White M (1995) Re-Authoring Lives: Interviews and Essays. Adelaide: Dulwich Centre Publications.

White W, Epston D (1990) Narrative Means to Therapeutic Ends. New York & London: Norton.

Williams A (1989) The Passionate Technique: Strategic Psychodrama with Individuals, Couples and Families. London & New York: Tavistock/Routledge.

Yalom I (1980) Existential Psychotherapy. New York, Basic Books.

Index

Printed and bound by CPI Group (UK) Ltd, Croydon, CR0 4YY

09/06/2025

14686002-0001